Children's Orthopaedics—
Practical Problems

Children's Orthopaedics—
Practical Problems

N. J. BLOCKEY, M.Ch.Orth., F.R.C.S. (Eng. and Glas.)

Barclay Lecturer in Orthopaedics, Glasgow University;
Consultant Orthopaedic Surgeon,
Royal Hospital for Sick Children, Glasgow

BUTTERWORTHS

LONDON · BOSTON

SYDNEY · WELLINGTON · DURBAN · TORONTO

THE BUTTERWORTH GROUP

ENGLAND

Butterworth & Co (Publishers) Ltd
London: 88 Kingsway, WC2B 6AB

AUSTRALIA

Butterworths Pty Ltd
Sydney: 586 Pacific Highway, NSW 2067
Also at Melbourne, Brisbane, Adelaide
and Perth

SOUTH AFRICA

Butterworth & Co (South Africa) (Pty) Ltd
Durban: 152–154 Gale Street

NEW ZEALAND

Butterworths of New Zealand Ltd
Wellington: 26–28 Waring Taylor Street

CANADA

Butterworth & Co (Canada) Ltd
Toronto: 2265 Midland Avenue,
  Scarborough, Ontario, M1P 4S1

USA

Butterworths (Publishers) Inc
Boston: 19 Cummings Park,
  Woburn, Mass. 01801

First published 1976

ISBN 0 407 00040 2

© Butterworth & Co (Publishers) Ltd 1976

Library of Congress Cataloging in Publication Data
Blockey, Noël Jackson.
    Children's orthopaedics.

    Bibliography: p.
    Includes index.
    1. Pediatric orthopedia. I. Title.
[DNLM: 1. Orthopedics—In infancy and childhood.
WS270 B687a]
RJ480.B56   617'.3   75–17552
ISBN 0–407–00040–2

Printed in Great Britain by
Butler & Tanner Ltd, Frome and London

Contents

Foreword

Sir Harry Platt Bt., LL.D., M.D., M.S., F.R.C.S., F.A.C.S.

Emeritus Professor of Orthopaedic Surgery, University of Manchester
Past President Royal College of Surgeons of England
Honorary President International Federation of Surgical Colleges

Mr Noël Blockey has always had the courage to expound his views on many of the debatable problems in the field of orthopaedics. During his formative years in the University Department of Orthopaedic Surgery in the Manchester Royal Infirmary, this quality, both to me as his Chief and to his contemporaries and juniors, was most stimulating. Now with the ripeness of years of experience in Glasgow at the Royal Hospital for Sick Children, Mr Blockey has selected a number of topics in which, with some justification, he feels that he has something of practical importance to convey to the postgraduate student of orthopaedics. As I read this collection of essays I recapture the essence of his critical mind, and I welcome the privilege of writing this foreword.

H. P.

Preface

My purpose in writing these essays is to give practical guidance to those in training on some of the problems they will meet. Current textbooks give comprehensive coverage of the whole field but fail to provide grounds for choosing one method of treatment from the many available. Ferguson (1968),* describing treatment of osteomyelitis, states, '... it may be treated and cured with the correct antibiotic, given a sufficiently long period of time to prevent recurrence...' This gives little help to the trainee who requires evidence to make his choice of drug and decide on length of treatment, and this I have tried to provide in my essay on osteomyelitis.

The other major essay is an attempt to steer a sensible course through the problems of congenital dislocation of the hip. A surgeon without a large personal series must know what results to expect from an exactly described course of treatment. End result studies of a collection of children treated differently help but little with decisions concerning management. It is to try to remedy these defects that the main essays have been written.

The other essays concern practical problems not, in my view, adequately covered elsewhere. This is because some, like haemarthrosis, have paediatric implications and others, like toe walking, appear to be new disorders. By giving personal experience ambiguity is avoided.

I apologize if I have been harshly critical of others but I do not retract any of my statements. Postgraduate discussion should be critical.

* Ferguson, A. B. (1968). *Orthopaedic Surgery in Infancy and Childhood* (3rd edn). Baltimore; Williams and Wilkins.

I am indebted to my colleagues both in orthopaedics and paediatrics with whom it has been a pleasure and a stimulus to work, to Mr Devlin and his staff for the photographic work and to Mrs Rita Miller and Miss Rose McColl for uncomplaining hours at the typewriter.

I am grateful to the Editor of *Journal of Bone and Joint Surgery* for permission to publish illustrations for the osteomyelitis essay that have previously appeared in that journal.

For the foreword it is a great pleasure to thank Sir Harry Platt. He first inspired me to follow this career and without his guidance over very many years I would not have had anything to say.

N J. Blockey

1 Minor Problems

The number of parents seeking orthopaedic consultations for their children is seemingly limitless. As the classic deformities are dealt with and infective and nutritional diseases eliminated one might expect fewer consultations from a given population. Affluence and greater parental care, however, nullify this trend. The numbers remain high but the problems are different. The older textbooks offer little guidance to the clinician facing children's orthopaedic clinics of today. Although the complaints seem trivial to the clinician they are worrying to the parents and must be carefully handled. To us the word 'normal' means 'not pathological' but to parents it means 'like the others'. The stature of the child often causes concern. We have to remember the wide normal variation. A boy aged 4 years may be anything from 93 cm to 110 cm and still be normal in our terms. There is a wide normal variation in foot size, in arch height and in the angles between the two feet for standing and walking. There are straight backs and round backs just as there is curly hair and straight hair. One has to adopt a reassuring role which is based on knowledge of the natural history of the deformity or ailment presenting. The vast number of these referrals is a reflection on the content of the undergraduate orthopaedic syllabus. We cannot expect the general practitioners to manage these minor problems themselves if we fail to teach or write about them.

This essay deals with three causes of concern to parents which are increasing in frequency: delay in walking, toe walking and small stature. More familiar conditions are then discussed where the textbooks give insufficient help to the clinician.

DELAY IN WALKING

The four commonest causes of significant delay in walking are congenital dislocation of the hip, flaccid paralysis, cerebral palsy of infancy and mental retardation. Exclusion of these conditions leaves
a large group of children for whom no obvious cause for delay can
be found. A history of how the baby first moved is important. There
are crawlers and shufflers. Ninety per cent of the human race crawl
on hands and knees before they pull themselves up into the standing
position. The 90th centile for independent walking of this 90 per cent
who crawl first is 15 months. Their preferred lying position is prone
and throughout infancy they have normal muscle tone. An affluent
society tends nowadays to provide baby walkers and baby bouncers
for its children in order presumably to advance the arrival of independent walking. These devices serve only to divert and entertain and
are of no orthopaedic value to the normal infant.

Ten per cent of the human race, however, do not crawl. They
shuffle or hitch themselves along on their bottoms. This 10 per cent
have characteristics not widely enough known among orthopaedic
surgeons. Their preferred lying position is supine, their musculature
is hypotonic, their motor development is delayed and 90 per cent
of them are not walking independently until 30 months of age. As
well as describing these features Robson (1970) has also shown a pure
dominant inheritance of shuffling in infancy: thus there is a 50 per
cent chance of shuffling among first degree relatives. These infants
are none the less normal. If they ever crawl it is with their knees
apart but they often simply get up and walk without any preliminary
crawling phase. The importance of distinguishing them from the
other 90 per cent of infants who crawl is partly to help to distinguish
the normal child of 24 months who is not walking from the abnormal
and partly to distinguish the condition from cerebral palsy, to
prevent physiotherapy being administered to the child and to avoid
confusion when a child with cerebral palsy is also a shuffler. In this
last situation the spasticity may be delayed. We have seen one such
child who propelled himself along on his back like a torpedo: muscle
tone was normal but the reflexes brisk.

TOE WALKING

The two commonest causes of a child walking on the toes are spastic
diplegia and peroneal muscular atrophy (Charcot–Marie–Tooth). In
recent years children have presented who are persistent toe walkers
without stigmata of chronic neurological or muscular disorder. They

present in the second year of life, the disorder is bilateral, they are otherwise healthy and the stance is normal. When they walk their feet assume an equinus position which is more marked on hurrying. Passively the feet can be brought up to a right angle without force. They have normal reflexes. In their history is often a period spent in a baby walker in which the infant from 6 months to 15 months has spent long periods. Such children appear to have the habit of toe walking imprinted on their motor development. The outlook is almost always good. The syndrome is new. We saw 11 such children in 1972 and 1973 but none in 1962–63 and the increased incidence in recent years is due to the common use nowadays of the 'baby walker'. Most children develop a normal gait when this device is abandoned. Occasionally it has been necessary to put the foot into plaster at right angles for 6 weeks. In one child in whom toe walking resumed after plaster fixation it was only cured by the wearing of wooden clogs.

One boy attended at age 8 years with a story of persistent toe walking from age one year. He had been extremely fond of his baby walker in which he spent long periods in infancy. After he had outgrown it, toe walking persisted but was disregarded. At school this boy, with a natural bounce in his gait, was directed to the dancing class. At this activity he excelled and it was not until after 3 years of this that advice was sought. His calves were organically shortened. With the knees flexed it was possible to put the foot almost at 90 degrees but on straightening the knee, tight equinus was evident and the gastrocnemius muscle was firm and bunched up. Apart from calf shortening there were no other features of neurological or muscular disease. Open elongation of the Achilles tendon was performed to put the foot at right angles. Histology of the calf muscle (*Figure 1.1*) showed 'floccular change of the sarcoplasm with swelling of nuclei. Increase of adipose tissue within muscle bundles and separating groups of fibres. Some fibres contained phagocytic cells. These changes are not diagnostic of any specific condition but are similar to changes seen in some non-progressive muscular dystrophies.' The operation was successful and at 1- and 2-year follow-ups he was within normal limits. I do not think this boy had or has any muscular dystrophy. The histology very closely resembles that reported by Cooper (1972) for a normal cat muscle immobilized in a shortened position for 22 weeks. It is thus likely that the unusual habits of this boy produced first voluntary contracture and then organic contracture.

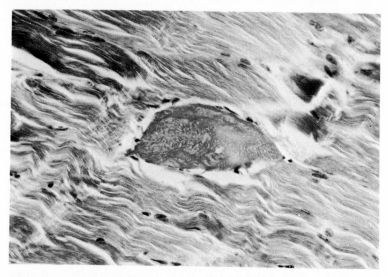

Figure 1.1. Muscle histology (× 125) from a persistent toe walker. Floccular change of the sarcoplasm (centre). Some fibres contain phagocytic cells. Changes suggestive of dystrophy

This may be the same condition described by Hall, Salter and Bhalla (1967) in 20 Canadian children. Seven of their children had biopsy examination and the muscle was reported to be normal. The presenting features suggested muscular dystrophy but no child turned out to have any organic diseases. The authors coin the term 'congenital short tendo-calcaneus' and as in my patient elongation of the tendo Achilles cured them. If this lesion were congenital it would be described in the neonatal period. I know of no experience or description of pure equinus deformity in the otherwise normal newborn. The evidence suggests that 'habitual calf contracture' would be a better diagnosis.

THE SMALL PATIENT

Ninety per cent of the boys who develop Perthes' disease are shorter and lighter than average for their age. Many other children attending orthopaedic outpatients are small for their age and the clinician is often asked for an explanation, a prognosis and a treatment.

If a child is above the third centile for height the smallness is un-likely at any age to be other than a normal variation.

A child below the third centile for height is likely to remain small and consistently below the average if his parents are small, i.e. father under 160 cm and mother under 145 cm (Queen Victoria's height) or he had a low birth weight. If the parents are normal one must establish when the smallness was first noticed. Primordial dwarfs have been small from the start and this will continue. There is no treatment. On the other hand smallness due to growth hormone defects have a definite starting point. Such statements as, 'He was normal up to age 3 years but I haven't had to buy him any bigger sized shoes since then' would suggest this cause. Investigations should follow before reference of the treatable cases to the endocrinologist. Radiographs of the wrist should be taken and compared with the Tanner Whitehouse scale. This can give an accuracy of 0.1 years. Retardation of bone age may be gross suggesting subthyroidism where epiphyseal dysgenesis would be expected. If retardation is not gross—say only 2 years behind the average for chronological age—further investigations should follow. The patient is admitted for growth hormone assay. The old investigations of assay of the protein-bound iodine and serum cholesterol have been superseded. On a fasting patient hypoglycalaemia is induced by the intravenous (iv) injection of 0.1 units of soluble insulin per kg bodyweight. Six samples of blood each sufficient to give 6 ml of serum are withdrawn at 30-minute intervals and submitted to biochemists for assay. From the results so obtained not only can growth hormone deficiency be established but hormonal deficiencies can be disclosed which might only become evident at puberty. If there is growth hormone deficiency it is now possible, provided anthropomorphic measurements and some longer term growth chart studies are confirmatory, to remedy the deficit. If growth hormone deficiency is not found anabolic steroids can be considered as a method of increasing height and weight.

It is not possible to tell by looking at the child whether there is or is not likelihood of growth hormone defect nor does IQ help as this is not hormone dependent.

It is not fruitful to pursue these investigations unless: (1) there is no obvious cause for the smallness; and (2) the child is below the third centile.

FLAT FOOT

Excluding vertical talus (congenital) flat foot of infants and peroneal spastic flat foot of teenagers there are two other age groups were flatness worries parents and the child's feet are fully mobile.

Aged 1–3 years

Over 90 per cent of children between the ages of 1 and 3 years with flat feet and oval footprints will improve spontaneously without specific treatment. Muscle tone develops in the invertors to bring about improvement. This applies also to those whose lateral radiographs

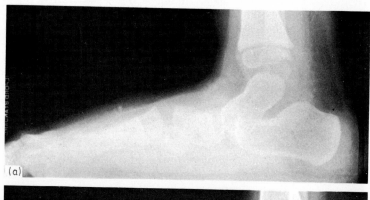

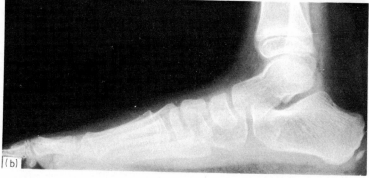

Figure 1.2. (a) Lateral weight-bearing radiograph of a child's foot at age 30 months. The arch is flat and the foot is valgus. This is not vertical talus flat foot. (b) Lateral radiograph of the same foot 6 years later. Without treatment the foot has become normal

show a more vertical disposition of the talus than expected (*Figure 1.2a*). Such a feature is invariable in valgus feet and should not persuade the clinician that he is dealing with a more serious lesion. If on tickling the sole of a young child's feet an arch appears as the foot is withdrawn then the outlook is good. The muscles are working and spontaneous improvement will occur (*Figure 1.2b*). The only exceptions are among the grossly overweight and the mentally retarded.

Aged 4–8 years

Long, thin narrow feet in young school children can cause concern. They present because they do not fit the parents' blueprint of normal. Such children are often tall and have recently had a growth spurt. They are not among the 10 per cent of infants who have failed to show spontaneous arch development by age 5 years. Their feet have not caused concern in the early years. Children in this group are non-ticklish. They walk in some external rotation, distort the inner wall of their shoes and wear down the inner side of sole and heel. There may be pain along the medial longitudinal arch. They are imprecise in their movements and while many can run fast they are beaten in acceleration and neatness by the others in this age group with straighter, shorter feet. Provided, as before, that they are not grossly overweight or otherwise afflicted they will improve spontaneously. This they do by beginning to put weight on the outer border of the foot and overcoming the external rotation. It may be necessary to initiate this development by advice to walk with their feet pointing directly forward, to walk on their toes a little each day and to stand at rest on the outer borders with the soles of the shoes resting against each other. They learn these exercises very quickly and it is exceptional for symptoms to persist longer than 1 year. The very small number who fail to develop this habit remain with an external rotation gait and progress to gross flatness though often without any symptoms. They grow into heavy, non-athletic teenagers somewhat ungainly in appearance and movement, requiring shoes which are bigger and which must be replaced more often than their parents consider normal.

INTOEING

Postural

A mild hen-toed gait in a toddler is within normal limits. The 'deformity' is often worsened by the child's habit of sitting on the feet or sleeping in the face down position. It will also be worsened by shoes with crooked and elongated heels or the Inneraze pattern. If the deformity is correctable passively, i.e. the first metatarsal can be placed in line with the medial border of the heel, improvement will occur if barefoot walking is encouraged and the child is dissuaded from the two rest positions just mentioned. Wearing shoes on the foot opposite to that intended is not necessary or desirable nor is a night external-rotation splint.

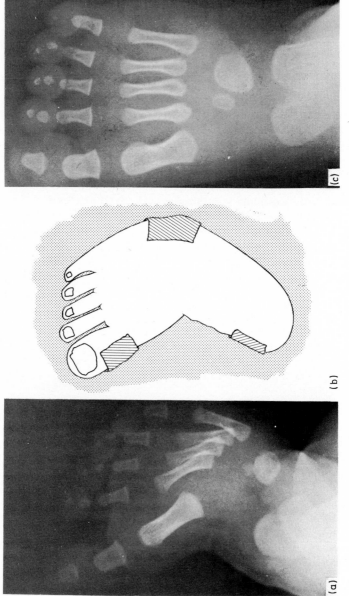

Figure 1.3. (a) Radiograph showing structural metatarsus varus in an infant. (b) Diagrammatic representation of the foot showing position of felt pads. (c) After repeated manipulation and plaster fixation normal alignment has been achieved and maintained

Structural

Metatarsus varus in an infant where the foot has a pronounced convexity to its outer edge will also show a deep sulcus medially. There is clinical and radiological evidence in such a foot of lateral displacement of the metatarsal bases associated with marked medial displacement of their heads (*Figure 1.3a*).

Such feet are variants of talipes equinovarus and must receive similar early and radical treatment.

Pads of adhesive felt are placed over the medial side of the first metatarsal head and neck, another over the base of the fifth metatarsal laterally and a third on the medial side of the heel (*Figure 1.3b*). A carefully moulded plaster is now applied, correcting the deformity by pushing the fifth metatarsal base medially while pulling the calcaneal region and the head of metatarsal 1 laterally. This is repeated at 2 weeks giving further opening of the inner concavity. *Figure 1.3c* shows the correction so achieved. If during these manipulations a resistant tight band is felt in the medial fasciculus of the plantar fascia this should be divided. Repeated manipulations may be necessary. Children so treated have some residual intoeing for which outer sole raises are used. The feet become acceptable and last for life without symptoms. Children who present with intoeing tend to have above average athletic ability.

KNOCK-KNEE AND BOW LEG

Figure 1.4 illustrates bow leg which is a common problem in child outpatients.

These three photographs portray Charles P. at age 11 months, 6 years and 15 years. Little can be added to their message.

Provided that rickets, either dietary or due to renal disease, can be excluded there is a very high spontaneous cure rate in these two conditions.

Bow leg begins to improve about 6 months after nappies are shed. If there is no improvement within a year of this event the baby may be either overweight or achondroplastic. The pre-school child with knock-knee should have the deformity measured by the space between the medial malleoli when standing with the knees touching. In otherwise healthy children all in the age group 2–5 years who have an intermalleolar separation of 3 inches or less will improve spontaneously in the following 2 years. It is the few whose improvement is incomplete and who are overweight who cause parental anxiety in older childhood. Among these few are the children who require

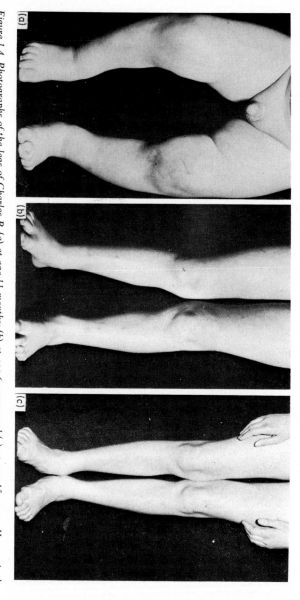

Figure 1.4. Photographs of the legs of Charles P. (a) at age 11 months; (b) at age 6 years; and (c) at age 15 years. He received no treatment

supracondylar femoral osteotomy at age 9–12 years. The infant who is obese at birth tends to have bow leg at age 1 year whereas the child whose birth weight is average but who is overweight at age 1 year can be expected to present at age $2\frac{1}{2}$–4 years with knock-knee. I know of no convincing evidence that crooked and elongated heels added to the shoes aids the spontaneous recovery in knock-knee. Any child with knock-knee and intoeing should be left untreated — the second deformity is the natural corrective for the former. The combination of knock-knee with flat foot often occurs in clumsy, big children who are non-ticklish and of poor athletic performance. They are helped by exercises which encourage weight to be borne on the outer edge of the foot as described earlier for flat foot.

INTERPHALANGEAL (IP) HALLUX VALGUS

The terminal phalanx lengthens by growth from a proximal epiphyseal plate which appears at age 2–4 years and fuses at age 18 years. In children who develop IP valgus this epiphyseal plate is bigger medially than laterally. As well as slight valgus a bony hard swelling is seen (*Figure 1.5*). This is, like a heel bump, thickened skin and fibrous tissue overlying an enlarged bone. It is not an exostosis. It cannot and should not be removed. Symptoms only arise from shoe pressure and friction and should be managed accordingly. Long-lasting disability is rare and function normal although slight flexion deformity develops accompanying the slight valgus.

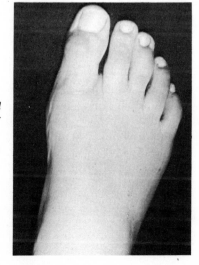

Figure 1.5. Interphalangeal valgus and pea-sized mass at age 11 years. Genetically determined epiphyseal deformity

CURLING TOES

Curled toes and toes on a different plane from their fellows are congenital deformities (*Figure 1.6*). They are not caused by but may be worsened by too tight socks and shoes. Such toes do not give rise to disability later in life, do not become hammer toes and need not be treated. They neither worsen nor improve. Radiographs show underdevelopment of the whole ray.

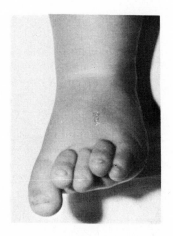

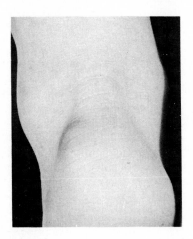

Figure 1.6. Curling toes at age 1 year. Genetically determined

Figure 1.7. Heel bump in a girl aged 12 years

HEEL BUMPS

Enlargement of the posterolateral corner of the calcaneum is common. Symptoms from such a minor congenital malformation can arise in schoolgirls because of constant friction between this enlargement and an ill-fitting shoe. The girl presents with thickened skin over the prominence (*Figure 1.7*). A callus forms. The disorder is bilateral and often wrongly termed an exostosis. Avoidance of the friction and the passage of time usually bring about improvement. If excision is performed the finding is thickened skin overlying a ridge of articular cartilage which is the posterolateral corner of the calcaneum. No exostosis is seen. Wedge osteotomy of the calcaneum is effective but should only be used after a prolonged trial of simpler measures.

OSGOOD–SCHLATTER'S DISEASE

Exploration and attempted removal of the painful hard swelling palpable just proximal to the broad insertion of the quadriceps muscle in teenage children usually contributes nothing. The swelling re-forms with equal tenderness and discomfort. This common event has caused further thought on aetiology and management. The disorder occurs in games-playing children aged 12–15 years. There is acute tenderness over the midline tibial swelling. Knee extension is not limited or painful. Direct pressure over the lump lying proximal

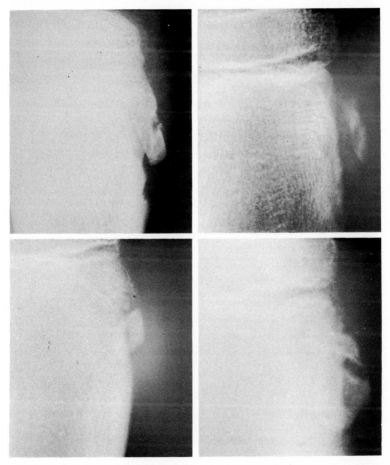

Figure 1.8. Lateral radiographs of the knee of 4 children aged 12–14 years with tenderness over the tibial tubercle. The tongue-like epiphysis is in two parts. The lesion is a fracture

to the quadriceps insertion is exquisitely painful. Radiographs show that the tongue-like epiphyseal prolongation is in two parts whereas that on the normal, painless side is not so split. These facts suggest that the lesion is a fracture of the tongue epiphysis due to kneeling or other direct violence. Avoidance of direct violence for 6 months or encasing the leg straight in a plaster cylinder both bring about resolution of the symptoms and signs and there is no recurrence. I believe the fragmentation so often described suggests a fracture rather than an 'osteochondritis' (*Figure 1.8*).

AMPUTATED FINGER TIP

The common injury produced when the tip of a toddler's finger is amputated by a closing drawer or a slammed door can be treated by thorough cleaning and sterile dressing. Even in cases where the terminal phalanx is exposed spontaneous healing will occur within 3 weeks. The result of such 'neglect' is attractive cosmetically. Flap closure after resection of bone, full thickness pedicle graft or split skin grafts are unnecessary and do not improve the results in the toddler.

MINOR PROBLEMS FOR THE SURGEON

No operator can claim that his year of theatre sessions has gone totally without anxiety. The complexity and unreliability of the equipment we use can land us in difficult situations. Fixation of osteotomy either subtrochanteric or humeral can go wrong in the best of hands. The author has extricated himself from difficult situations by realizing that the round-bodied Blount stainless steel staple now largely superseded by the vitallium reinforced angle staple will give a satisfactory press fit into accurately drilled holes of $\frac{3}{32}$ inch diameter (No. 43). This avoids the need to hammer the staple home which too often moves the osteotomy.

REFERENCES

Cooper, R. R. (1972). *J. Bone Jt Sturg.* **54A,** 919
Hall, J. E., Salter, R. B. and Bhalla, S. K. (1967). *J. Bone Jt Surg.* **49B,** 695
Robson, P. (1970). *Developmental Medicine and Child Neurology* **12,** 608

2 Osteomyelitis

OSTEOMYELITIS

Those who have had to treat osteomyelitis in the past are only too aware of features of the disease which today can be regarded as rare and largely preventable complications. They regularly encountered sequestration and intra-osseous abscess and sinus formation. Less commonly, but none the less disastrously, there were the complications of pyogenic arthritis, pathological fracture, epiphyseal growth plate destruction, metastatic bacterial infection and, last, the dreaded amyloid disease.

Today all these are avoidable with correct management of the acute disease. This chapter discusses avoidance of these complications and their treatment where avoidance has failed.

Successful management entails early diagnosis and correct decisions regarding the choice of antibiotics, the place of surgery and the duration of treatment. Whilst vast strides have been made in chemotherapy in the last 20 years the large number of available antibiotics makes choice difficult. The clinician must steer a middle course between using only drugs with which he is familiar and the alternative of using the drug whose promotion literature was last placed on his desk.

Although complications are rare in Britain today, they are common overseas. In spite of the considerable modern literature on the use of antibiotics some clinicians still delay treatment until they have cultured the organism. Some use agents like intravenous tetracycline for septicaemia, and fail to adjust the choice or dosage of antibiotic to the needs of the clinical problem. We cannot avoid the complications of this disease without eradicating these errors.

Choice of antibiotic

Three years ago a paper concerning the choice of antibiotics in this disease was published (Blockey and McAllister, 1972). The authors defined acute osteomyelitis as an inflammation of bone of sudden onset caused by pyogenic organisms in the bloodstream, their presence in the blood being proved and/or their effects on the bone demonstrated by specific radiographic changes. Success of primary treatment was accepted when the signs and symptoms were cured within 4 weeks of first admission to hospital and no complications of the local bone disease developed thereafter.

Over a 12-year period various antibiotics were compared. The highest success rate among the combinations tested was 89.5 per cent in 38 proven cases in which fusidic acid combined with either benzyl-penicillin or erythromycin was used depending on staphylococcal sensitivity.

Fusidic acid was chosen to follow the cloxacillin–benzylpenicillin series because evidence showed increasing prevalence of benzyl-penicillin-resistance among invading staphylococci and it was thought likely that cloxacillin-resistance would develop in similar fashion.

This predicted change towards cloxacillin-resistance among sta-phylococci has not proved to be widespread in the United Kingdom. Whilst the figures for staphylococcal sensitivity to benzylpenicillin are now 10.3 per cent for inpatients and 8.8 per cent for outpatients (McAllister, 1975) our figures for cloxacillin-resistance in 1973 were 1.0 per cent for inpatients and 0.2 per cent for outpatients. Reports of higher resistance to cloxacillin from elsewhere, i.e. Jensen and Lassen (1969) and Ridley et al. (1970) appear to be local outbreaks of multiply-resistant strains with a high cross-infection rate. The success rate in 55 consecutive proven cases using benzylpenicillin and cloxacillin was 85.5 per cent using cloxacillin in a dose of 1 g/day for a child aged under 12 years. We now believe that we were under-treating some of these children and the success rate might have been higher on a dose of 5 g/day. Should we therefore now give an extended trial to cloxacillin in a dose of 5–10 g/day? To be able to use the intramuscular route is a big advantage over fusidic acid in the very young and the very ill.

The management of two comparable series differing only in the antibiotic used showed 14.5 per cent failure with cloxacillin (1 g/day) as against 10.5 per cent for fusidic acid (30 mg/kg/day). Seven of the 8 failures in the cloxacillin group were in children with staphylo-coccal disease of the long bones but there were no failures among those with the same conditions in the fusidic acid series. Further-more, incomplete healing was present after 21 days' therapy in 42 of 113 children given antibiotics other than fusidic acid and 7 of this group flared up. In the fusidic acid series 3 of 38 showed incomplete healing after 21 days' therapy and none flared up. Experience from May 1972—the end of the fusidic acid series previously reported—confirms that, of the antibiotics tested, fusidic acid is the most effective. We see no point in changing. Fusidic acid and erythromycin stearate each in a dose of 30 mg/kg/day in 4 divided doses is now recommended for a child aged under 12 years. In the seriously ill and the very young we find oral dosage unreliable and recommend cloxacillin 100 mg/kg/day by intramuscular injection for the first 48 hours followed by the fusidic acid/erythromycin regime unless bacteriological reports suggest otherwise. Should the organism prove to be *Haemophilus influenzae* (expected incidence 2.5 per cent, but perhaps growing) we change to ampicillin 100 mg/kg/day by injection.

Effective tissue levels

Fusidic acid levels in pus and living and dead bone were recorded in patients under treatment (Blockey and McAllister, 1972) and found to be effective. Deodhar *et al.* (1972) have shown effective synovial levels in diseased joints on oral fusidic acid, whereas with cloxacillin we can find no such evidence. Unpublished work in adults (Jones, 1974) suggests that a dose of 500 mg 6-hourly would give just adequate serum and bone levels but a dose of 250 mg 6-hourly plus 500 mg 1 hour before removing the specimens would not. We await published work to support the clinical impression that parenteral cloxacillin is effective in early staphylococcal bone disease. In one of our children aged 9 years and of weight 30 kg an oral dose of 1 g cloxacillin 6-hourly gave a serum level of 10.5 μg/ml 1 hour after the dose but 5 hours later the serum contained trace amounts only. In another patient (weight 28 kg) with a serious femoral neck infection an oral dose of 5 g/day was given for 6 weeks. At operation during the third week an intra-osseous abscess was opened and no cloxacillin was detected in the pus. Another patient aged 9 years had a tibial bone abscess explored $3\frac{1}{2}$ hours after an intramuscular (im) dose of 1 g of cloxacillin and pus from the cavity showed a cloxacillin level of 1.9 μg/ml. The use of flucloxacillin instead of cloxacillin halves the dosage required but does not prolong the effective serum level beyond about 3 hours.

Parenteral therapy

A severely ill child with or without vomiting should receive intramuscular cloxacillin in a dose of 100 mg/kg/day in divided doses 4-hourly. If there is also fluid depletion intravenous therapy should be given. We have reported successes with diethanolamine fusidate (Blockey and McAllister, 1972) but reports of tissue levels after cloxacillin are rare. In one patient (weight 32 kg) an iv transfusion of half-strength saline in 5 per cent dextrose containing 2 g cloxacillin/500 ml of fluid was set up and delivered at 42 ml/hour, i.e. 500 ml in 12 hours. Serum cloxacillin levels in this boy were:

After 4 hours	16 μg/ml
After 8 hours	24 μg/ml
After 24 hours	19 μg/ml

This suggests that iv fluid containing 4 g cloxacillin/litre for 24 hours gives continuous effective serum levels of antibiotic which are higher than those achieved 1 hour after an oral dose of 1 g in a patient of the same size. It is fair to assume that bone levels are related to serum levels but published work on this point is lacking. It is sometimes argued that peak serum levels are best achieved by administering cloxacillin by the 'bolus' method, i.e. 1 g/20 ml 6-hourly, rather than by a continuous infusion. We have no evidence to support this.

Treatment of septicaemia

On clinical diagnosis of septicaemia in an ill child with no guide to causative organism a cephalosporin (cephaloridine, cephalothin, cephradine or cephazolin) or an aminoglycoside (gentamicin, tobramycin) should be given intravenously after blood culture (McAllister, 1975). There is no way of telling in a desperate situation whether the infection is Gram-positive or Gram-negative and thus a parenteral broad-spectrum antibiotic is required.

Consideration of other antibiotics

We are sometimes criticized for not using other antibiotics which we are told might improve results. There is insufficient time in a clinical lifetime to test all the possibilities. One must first treat a significant number of proven cases, perhaps 30 or more; then these must be followed up until there is a strong likelihood that reactivations of infection which are going to occur have done so—nothing short of 2 years will do. Thus, to get comparable data would take 4 years even in a hospital accepting 15 proven cases each year. If one accepts 'clinical' cases, i.e. those without specific radiographic changes and with negative blood cultures, it would be easy to make the diagnosis in 30 children in any one year, but by so doing the successful result percentage would be of less value. To be swayed in favour of another antibiotic combination I would require an analysis of proven bone infections in children using similar definitions to those I have quoted.

To establish the best-guess antibiotic combination one has to predict the causal organisms. There is very little variation here between one series and another. Acute osteomyelitis in children is caused by:

Staphylococcus aureus	86–90 per cent
Streptococcus pyogenes	4–7 per cent
Haemophilus influenzae	2–4 per cent
Salmonellae	
Escherichia coli	1–2 per cent
Proteus	

McAllister (1975) has measured the sensitivity of 1271 strains of *Staph. aureus* obtained from inpatients in 3 hospitals to 10 antibiotics in common use in staphylococcal infections. His figures in order of superiority are: gentamicin 100 per cent sensitive; co-trimoxazole 99.6 per cent; cloxacillin 99.0 per cent; cephaloridine 99.0 per cent; lincomycin 98.9 per cent; neomycin 98.4 per cent; fusidic acid 98.1 per cent; erythromycin 94.6 per cent; tetracycline 76.9 per cent; benzylpenicillin 10.3 per cent. With the causative organisms recognized the agents to use would be among these 10. There are strong advocates of at least the first 8.

Some writers have advised waiting for bacteriological proof of the infecting agent but in clinical practice one-third of blood cultures from patients thought by responsible clinicians to have acute osteomyelitis will be negative. Furthermore, even with expert laboratory assistance the specimens cannot be subcultured until 18 hours after collection, giving the minimum time for a positive culture 36 to 42 hours and sensitivity testing another 18 to 24 hours. A delay of this duration in an urgent clinical situation is inexcusable.

Considering the *H. influenzae* infections, whose incidence seems to be rising slightly (6 per cent in the series 1969/70), McAllister (1975) found the following percentage sensitivities, testing 66 strains against 7 antibiotics. Ampicillin 100 per cent sensitive; tetracycline 100 per cent; erthromycin 98.8 per cent, cephaloridine 94.2 per cent; co-trimoxazole 89.7 per cent; benzylpenicillin 19.8 per cent; and lincomycin 0 per cent. Our experience with fusidic acid and erythromycin in the 3 years following our report of their use in 38 consecutive proven cases has been entirely satisfactory, and their use in acute osteomyelitis is still recommended. We do not, however, deny the others a place.

Benzylpenicillin is indicated in acute osteomyelitis where the infecting organism is known to be *Strep. pyogenes*, *Strep. pneumoniae* or the now rare *Staph. aureus* sensitive to benzylpenicillin. Tetracycline we have used once in recent years. The child was admitted with a large upper thigh abscess which was opened and yielded *H. influenzae.* She developed a metastatic pneumonia and was at the same time known to be hypersensitive to penicillin, thus ruling out ampicillin. The choice in this difficult situation lay between tetracycline and chloramphenicol; in spite of its tooth-staining properties the former was selected with success. Chloramphenicol has only one place in this disease—the infant with a proven *Strep. pneumoniae* infection who develops signs of meningitis. As benzylpenicillin is relatively poor at crossing the blood–brain barrier, chloramphenicol should be used. Apart from these rare exceptions neither of these should play any part in the treatment of osteomyelitis. Gentamicin would be likely to give good results in this disease but we consider its antistaphylococcal properties inferior to those of fusidic acid or cloxacillin and ototoxicity has been reported with high dosage (Jackson and Arcieri, 1971). It would not be our first-line choice unless a Gram-negative infection was proved. We have used it successfully in a case of osteomyelitis secondary to an implanted foreign body from which *Pseudomonas aeruginosa* was cultured. Co-trimoxazole (Septrin, Burroughs Welcome; Bactrim, Roche), reported effective in osteomyelitis in children from Uganda (Craven, Pugsley and Blowers, 1970), has been less well tolerated in our patients than its competitors. It lacks a parenteral form and is not suitable for the very young. We have used it effectively in a streptococcal infection where allergy to penicillin was thought likely. Cephaloridine (Ceporin, Glaxo) has the correct spectrum and is effective parenterally with good penetration; cephalexin (Ceporex, Glaxo; Keflex, Lilly) is the oral equivalent. Walker (1973) describes its use in 14 infants and children with acute osteomyelitis. The follow-up of 1–3 months is considered inadequate. Smith (1971) reported improvement in 4 out of 5 cases of osteomyelitis from Iowa after cephaloridine treatment. Larger series are awaited. We have used cephaloridine in an atypical infection in a small child thought to be allergic to penicillin. Lincomycin has been largely replaced by the better absorbed clindamycin (Dalacin C, Upjohn). This would be useless in *H. influenzae* infections and its recommendation in staphylococcal or streptococcal infections would require a more palatable oral form and more evidence of its efficacy in acute osteomyelitis. The pseudomembranous colitis recently reported (*Br. med. J.*, 1974) is worrying.

For pseudomonas infections gentamicin or tobramycin would be the drug of choice.

Unusual clinical problems

Obscure cases occur from time to time. Osteomyelitis of the spine or pelvis has presented in 5 children as pyrexia of unknown origin.

Others have had illnesses associated with radiographic evidence of bone disease in a surgically inaccessible site. For these children repeated blood cultures are necessary. We know of no way of predicting the optimum time. When all attempts to culture an organism fail the clinician must consider assay of antistaphylococcal antibody titres (Lack and Towers, 1962). However, reports suggest that the level of any of the four antibodies—antialphatoxin, antileucocidin, anticoagulase and antistaphylokinase—can be raised in normal children. The levels can also be normal in children proved to have staphylococcal disease. The techniques of assay are difficult and in our experience assessment of the result of a short trial of a potent antistaphylococcal antibiotic has been more useful in diagnosis.

Results of treatment of acute osteomyelitis in children

In the 10-year period of 1960–70, 151 proven cases were treated. Operation was performed only when there was clinical evidence of an abscess. Seventy-five such operations were performed and culture of the pus obtained yielded pathogenic organisms in 68. All the 75 children requiring operation had circulating antibiotics at the time of surgery.

The results in these 151 children—follow-up now 4–14 years—are:

Complete resolution of infection without cavity
    formation 88   126
Infected cavity on the 21-day radiograph   resolves 38   successes

                    45

Infected cavity on the 21-day radiograph   flare-ups   7
Developed sinus after 21 days 5   25
Sequestrum formation—chronicity or further spread 13   failures

           Total proven cases 151

The failure rate of primary treatment was therefore 16.6 per cent. Many differing antibiotics were used and the duration of treatment was not consistent in the early years. All the children had disease of the limb bones satisfying the definitions given. Infections of face, spine and pelvis were excluded. The sites of infection, the ages of the children involved, the length of history and the annual prevalences have been described (Blockey and Watson, 1968). Comparisons of various antibiotics and discussions on the duration of treatment occur in a later paper (Blockey and McAllister, 1972).

We must now discuss why failures of primary treatment occur and how they are managed.

Patterns of failure of primary treatment

Failures of treatment of acute osteomyelitis take two forms. There can be a gratifying clinical response to the antibiotics given but after 21 days of such therapy there are cavities either central or metaphyseal on the radiograph. These may appear quiescent, only to reactivate later. Failures also occur (*see* Chronic Osteomyelitis), where the incision, designed to drain pus from subperiosteal and intra-osseous areas, does not heal or breaks down after temporary healing and continues to discharge. These two clinical problems must be separated because the former may heal; the latter will not.

The infected cavity problem

If one treats all cases presenting at hospital with bedrest, splintage and effective antibiotics for 21 days, reserving operation for those showing clinical evidence of an abscess (about 50 per cent) there are three possible results. A large majority will be clinically normal; their radiographs will show slight periosteal elevation or minor cortical blemishes where the disease has been. *Figure 2.1* is a typical example. There will be some in whom failure of primary treatment has declared itself by sequestrum formation, wound breakdown and sinuses or continuing clinical disease. There will be a third group lying in between. These children will be improved compared with their condition on admission but their sedimentation rate may be raised and radiographs will show metaphyseal cavities (*Figures 2.3a* and *2.4a*).

The action the clinician should take poses a problem not encountered in the pre-antibiotic era. It could be argued (Spink, 1956; Schandling, 1960) that these cavities contain viable pathogens that antibiotics have failed to reach and operation should be performed. It could also be argued that these cavities contain the residuum of the infection and require more prolonged antibiotic treatment (Green, 1962). Thirdly, one could justify doing nothing on the grounds that once the clinical state has improved the child's own defences can be left to deal with the residual metaphyseal lesions. Clearly if this third course were justified the children would be saved both an operation and a further stay in hospital. To decide this question rationally demands a knowledge of whether those residual cavities do or do not contain pathogenic organisms.

A girl aged 8 years was treated for acute osteomyelitis of the lower tibia. After 21 days of treatment her sedimentation rate had fallen from 24 to 15 mm in the first hour. The radiographs showed ill-defined blemishes in the lower tibial metaphysis. The best delineation of these was on a 7 cm tomograph (*Figure 2.2*).

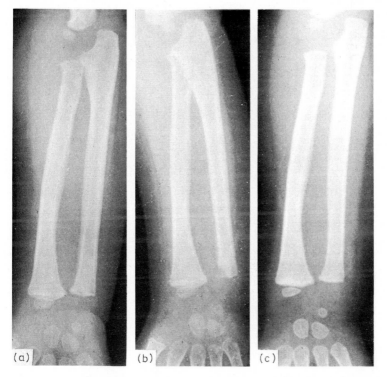

Figure 2.1. Radiographic progress of a lower ulnar lesion in a girl aged 4 years treated with fucidin and erythromycin. On diagnosis (a) there is no bone change, at 10 days (b) the lesion is seen and at 2 months the lesion has healed leaving no trace (c)

(By courtesy *J. Bone Jt Surg.,* 1970)

This case was selected because her erythrocyte sedimentation rate (ESR) was borderline and the radiographic changes, though not as marked as some others in this group, were present. Multiple drill holes were inserted into the metaphysis and culture of the contents grew *Staph. aureus* resistant to benzylpenicillin as had the blood culture on admission.

In spite of this evidence it was decided to observe cases presenting this problem in the hope of learning which were those that required treatment either by operation or further antibiotics.

The results table shows that 45 children were in this situation after 21 days of effective antibiotics. No treatment was given.

Figures 2.3 and 2.4 are radiographs from patients in this group. They were followed up for a minimum of 4 years and 38 of the 45

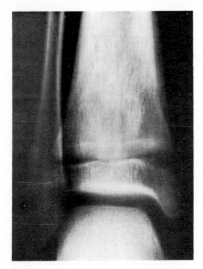

Figure 2.2. Anteroposterior tomograph of lower tibial lesion after 21 days of antibiotic treatment

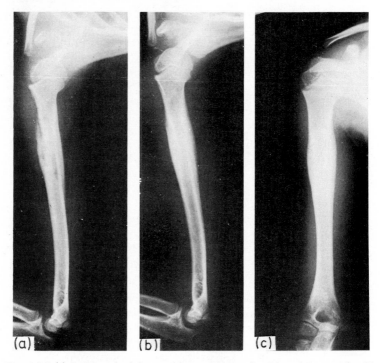

(a) (b) (c)

Figure 2.3. (a) Radiograph of the upper humeral lesion of a girl aged 6 years after 21 days of antibiotics for acute osteomyelitis. (b and c) Without treatment the lesion gradually healed over the course of 2 years

(By courtesy *J. Bone Jt Surg.,* 1970)

healed these lesions gradually over 2 years whereas the other 7 developed further extension of the metaphyseal disease requiring surgical treatment. The healing in the 38 children was symptomless. *Figures 2.3b and 2.4b* show the end result without treatment of the lesions shown in *2.3a* and *2.4a*. It seems, therefore, that about 7 of the 45 such lesions will give further trouble whereas the rest (5 out of 6) will heal. We found that the factor of greatest importance in deciding the likely outcome was the clinical state of the child after 21 days' therapy. Study of the radiographs did not show any differences between those settling and those flaring. An elevated sedimentation rate (about 15 mm in the first hour) was found in 17 of

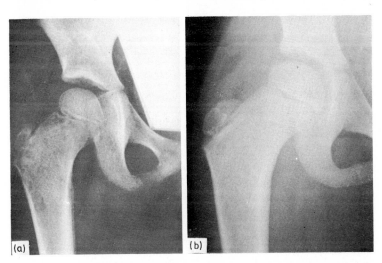

Figure 2.4. (a) *Anteroposterior radiographs of the right hip of a girl aged $4\frac{1}{2}$ years after 21 days of antibiotics for acute osteomyelitis.* (b) *Without treatment and following normal activities the lesions healed without trace within 2 years*

these children of which 14 resolved and 3 flared up, whereas of 8 whose ESR was normal, 7 healed and 1 did not. By clinical state is meant the range of movement in the neighbouring joint, the child's use of the limb and the effect of palpation. Where there were no physical signs in the limb after 21 days the infected cavities did not flare up, whereas in all children where flare-up occurred there was deep bony tenderness over the lesions although in many the joint movement was full. I have neither produced nor seen elsewhere any evidence that suggests that prolonging the antibiotic therapy beyond 21 days will significantly lessen the flare-up rate. Thus, it is now my policy to operate on localized accessible lesions which at 21 days *show physical signs* and radiographic evidence of metaphyseal cavities. Antibiotics are also continued. Those without deep tenderness and joint limitation are left alone. Operation will reveal the nature of the infection if not already known at this stage. If the lesion is staphylococcal antibiotics proved to have maximum penetration in diseased bone should be used. Fusidic acid combined with clindamycin is recommended. In inaccessible lesions where the organism is not known a combination of fusidic acid and erythromycin for a further 21 days is sensible. A cephalosporin (*see above*) should also be considered if a Gram-negative infection is possible.

CHRONIC OSTEOMYELITIS

This term refers to osteomyelitis with sequestra and abscesses resulting from failure of bacteriological cure of the acute lesion. It is rare in Britain but common overseas. The literature pays scant attention to the problem in children. Rowling (1969) treated 29 patients with radical surgery and fusidic acid therapy but only 1 was a child with a follow-up of 10 months. Maudsley and Taylor (1970) developed and reported an irrigation technique in 12 patients but only 1 was a child. My experience is of 13 children with follow-up of 6 years or more. All were healed by 1 year and have remained healed. These 13 had two factors in common: the management of the original infection was poor and the disease was staphylococcal.

Avoidance of chronicity

The correct management of the acute lesion is the best insurance against chronicity. This demands early diagnosis. To this end the classic teaching cannot be improved upon. Pain, swelling and loss of function with tenderness over the metaphysis are the cardinal signs. Pyrexia with raised sedimentation rate and leucocytosis are also present. Radiographs are normal for at least 10 days from the first symptoms and longer when the infection is in the femoral neck. These clinical features demand admission to an orthopaedic unit, rest of the affected limb in removable splintage and the start of effective antibiotic therapy after withdrawing blood samples for culture. Examination of the failures in our hands shows deviations from these principles.

> One girl was admitted with unexplained fever when she developed pain and tenderness in the lower femur with an effusion into the knee joint. She was given aspirin and local heat on a diagnosis of acute rheumatism. Another child was given cloxa-

cillin, 1 g/day in divided dosage for a probable acute infection of the femoral neck. When the blood culture showed *Streptococcus pyogenes* the clinician continued the cloxacillin in the same dosage, failing to realize that since cloxacillin is only about one-eighth as potent as benzylpenicillin 4.8 g cloxacillin would equate with 1 mega-unit (600 mg) benzylpenicillin. Two young children have been seen in isolation hospitals where the pseudo-paralysis, almost pathognomonic of acute osteomyelitis complicated by septic arthritis, was thought to be due to a virus infection.

In some children early operation, thought by some to be beneficial in this disease, has not been supported by adequate antibiotic therapy and sequestration has occurred. In most children where disease becomes chronic the mismanagement has been due to delay at home; their clinical signs have been ignored and they have only been admitted to hospital when the disease is advanced. It is the extent of the disease present when effective antibiotics are begun that decides the outcome. This is not consistently correlated with the length of history. Table 2.1 shows the results in 113 consecutive cases.

TABLE 2.1

Length of history	Cases	Failures
Less than 48 hours	32	3
2–5 days	51	12
6–14 days	27	6
Over 14 days	3	0

Management of lesions with sinus and sequestra

Figure 2.5a is the radiograph of the left humerus of a girl aged 8 years. She had been given benzylpenicillin and tetracycline for an infection found to be resistant to both drugs and 6 months after the onset of infection she had 3 sinuses. After admission and general medical care, cloxacillin 2 g/day in divided dosage was begun. Misjudgement in an earlier case had taught that sequestrectomy should be delayed until a strong involucrum had formed (*see Figure 2.25*). *Figures 2.5b–d* show progress in the first year of treatment. Lower sequestrectomy was performed at 5 months and upper sequestrectomy at 9 months. *Figure 2.5d* shows the bone after these two operations, at each of which extensive and careful removal of all infective tissue was carried out. The patient received cloxacillin 2 g/day for 2 months. This

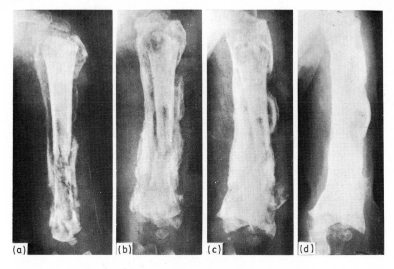

Figure 2.5. Chronic staphylococcal osteomyelitis in a girl aged 8 years. Radiographs taken every 3 months for 1 year

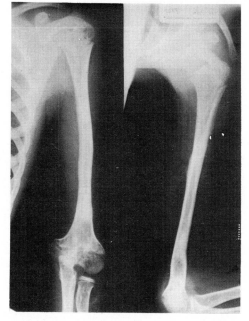

Figure 2.6. Radiographs of the same arm as in Figure 2.5, 5 years later. There is healing with remodelling

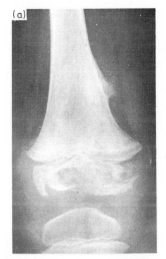

Figure 2.7. (a) is an anteroposterior radiograph of a painful swollen knee with two sinuses. (b) and (c) show the same joint 2 and 6 years later

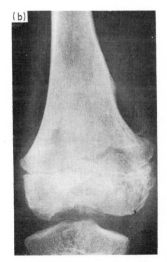

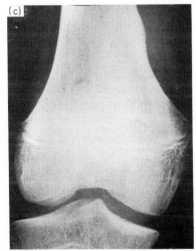

was repeated for each operation. The wounds healed and remained healed. *Figure 2.6* shows the arm at age 13 years. There has been beautiful remodelling and slight loss of carrying angle is the only permanent result of the infection.

Another example of success by following the principles laid down by Rowling for adults was a boy aged 4 years who on admission wore a caliper protecting a painful warm knee held at 20 degrees. There were two discharging sinuses just proximal to the joint line (*Figure 2.7a*). The boy had had seven previous operations and three courses of antibiotics in the previous 2 years.

At operation the whole cavity was laid open from the medial side leaving a mere shell of articular cartilage and bone. The scrapings cultured *Staph. aureus* resistant to benzylpenicillin. Complete evacuation of all infected tissue was achieved and 2 g cloxacillin was left in the cavity. The patient received oral cloxacillin 4 g daily for 6 weeks. The lesion healed and the cavity reossified. *Figure 2.7b* and *c* show the lesion 2 and 6 years later, respectively.

Fusidic acid is now replacing cloxacillin in the management of chronic osteomyelitis. Results are encouraging but there are no 6-year follow-up results to report. Repeated operations are necessary in this condition because of recurrent abscesses. Complete healing will not occur until all sequestra surrounded by infected tissue are removed with that infected tissue. Pathological fracture markedly worsens the outlook for the limb. The classic operation of diaphysectomy is useful if the affected bone can be spared.

The place of surgery in management of acute osteomyelitis

The commonest site in children is the lower femur. *Figure 2.8* shows the lower third of a normal femoral shaft at age 4 years in coronal section. This photograph shows the relative thickness of cortex, the absence of a medullary 'cavity' and uniform consistency of the marrow. Acute osteomyelitis is caused by multiplication of pyogenic bacteria in this tissue. Those who believe in 'early surgical drainage' for this disease should bear in mind the nature of the ground upon which they tread. I believe operation should only be performed when there is clinical evidence of an abscess. Fluctuation and localization should be searched for daily; hence the need for removable splintage. This is detected by palpating a soft area in the centre of induration at a bone end. Fluctuation always means that there is pus beneath the periosteum and is an absolute indication for operation. There is never any harm in waiting for these signs of localization of the infection. Pus may be clinically detectable on admission or may never form if antibiotic treatment is adequate and early. Timetable regimes are useless. Operations performed before subperiosteal pus has formed, designed to prevent bone destruction, have, in my hands, been disappointing. Seventy-five operations were performed in the series of 151 consecutive cases previously reported. All opened and evacuated subperiosteal abscesses. In none of these was pus found under pressure. Pus welled up into the wound—spurting was not seen. Spread to the subperiosteal area represents decompression of the metaphyseal lesion. The nidus of infection does not enter the medullary 'cavity' in childhood osteomyelitis because no cavity exists. In operations where, in addition to evacuation of the subperiosteal abscess, drill holes have been inserted into the metaphyseal

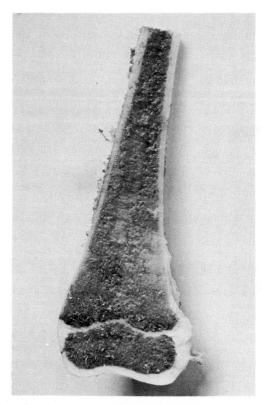

Figure 2.8. Coronal section of a normal lower femur at age 4 years

region and bacteriological culture taken from the central contents, these cultures have proved positive for the same organism and in the same proportion of cases as the subperiosteal pus. This suggests that decompression is natural and also suggests that metaphyseal drill holes will evacuate more pus than simply opening the subperiosteal space, thereby aiding the natural decompression and improving the access of the antibiotics.

Operation is also indicated when an adequate course of effective antibiotics has failed to render the lesion clinically and radiologically healed.

Surgical removal of any sequestrum surrounded by pus is always necessary. The exceptions occur in infants where simple evacuation of the abscess seems sufficient. Sequestra not surrounded by pus but nevertheless representing pieces of the original bone will, in children, become incorporated in the new bone as healing proceeds. *Figure 2.10b* and *c* show this process. Perhaps sequestra is the wrong name for them as their maintenance of normal architecture and their later incorporation suggests they behave exactly as do bone grafts in that they allow new bone to form on their surface. Pieces of original cortex isolated from the new bone by pus or granulation tissue have to be removed no matter how small. I know of no case where even a very small isolated sequestrum has become incorporated. If sequestrectomy is indicated the operation should be delayed until there is sufficient involucrum for stability of the limb to be maintained after surgery.

The case against early surgery

The arguments advanced by those who practise early, i.e. prophylactic, surgery, are based on the assumption that operation before an abscess is formed releases pressure and thus minimizes vascular damage. Their claim is that by operating early:

(1) the diagnosis is confirmed and the organism is obtained for sensitivity tests;

(2) vascular damage and bone necrosis are prevented or reduced to a minimum;

(3) pain relief is dramatic.

As this is a disease caused by predictable bacteria, it seems unnecessary to know their exact identity. A scar on a child's limb is too high a price to pay for bacteriological certainty. Operation will be a tragic mistake unless the infective lesion is found and evacuated. In adults a point of maximum tenderness can usually be found, but in children localization is difficult. An ill child with a tense swelling of the whole limb segment does not reveal the site of primary involvement. Two examples show this difficulty in localization. They are selected because in each case the wrong bone would have been explored if the policy of prophylactic operation had been followed.

A girl aged 2 years was admitted with intense pain and swelling in the left arm from mid-humeral level to the wrist. She had suffered for 4 days with increasing pain and disuse. Her radiograph showed severe soft-tissue swelling but no bony

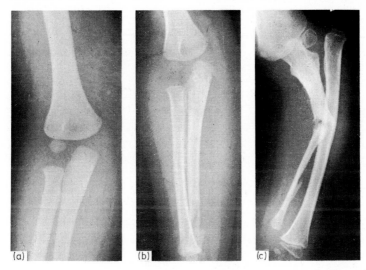

Figure 2.9. This girl shows the difficulty in localizing the disease at an early stage and also in predicting the outcome

involvement (*Figure 2.9a*). The diagnosis was lower humeral osteomyelitis. At 14 days radiographic and clinical evidence disclosed the infection in the ulnar shaft—an unusual site which led to serious complications (*Figure 2.9b and c*).

A second girl was admitted with a 2-day history of pain and uselessness of the left elbow and forearm. Radiographs were normal (*Figure 2.10a*). She was given benzylpenicillin and tetracycline and rested in a collar and cuff sling. She did not improve and 2 days later the swelling was maximal over the lower end of the ulna. Fluctuation was not detected. She was changed to methicillin. She improved and subsequent radiographs showed that it was the radial shaft that was involved (*Figure 2.10b*). A small abscess over the lower radius was drained and 4 years later (*Figure 2.10c*) the radiographs showed a normal appearance.

In both these cases, early operation, if performed, would have been on the wrong bone.

The clinical problem one faces is shown in *Figure 2.11*. A boy aged 8 years with a 3-day history of pain was admitted after being given benzylpenicillin for 'cellulitis'. Experience emphatically suggests that this boy should receive effective antibiotics after blood culture and not operative surgery.

Strict adherence to the policy advised by Harris (1962) will lead to unnecessary and useless operations. There can be no certain way

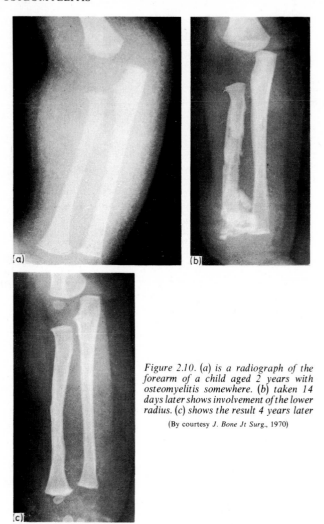

Figure 2.10. (a) is a radiograph of the forearm of a child aged 2 years with osteomyelitis somewhere. (b) taken 14 days later shows involvement of the lower radius. (c) shows the result 4 years later

(By courtesy J. Bone Jt Surg., 1970)

of knowing where the disease lies until it localizes. The lesion may heal under antibiotics or may progress to form an abscess. All such abscesses are extra-osseous and give the physical sign of fluctuation in the centre of an area of tender induration. This is an indication for operation. Opening will relieve pain and prevent possible skin necrosis and sinus formation. All such operations will produce pus. None will be useless.

It is now necessary to consider whether early operation (i.e. within 48 hours or before abscess formation) done on the correct site, is in fact useful. Is the pressure concept of pathology held by the advocates of early surgery correct? Does operation prevent vascular damage and bone necrosis?

Trueta (1957) has been the strongest advocate of early surgery. He, Larsen (1934) and Harris (1962) look upon the metaphyseal abscess as the primary focus. They argue that if this is not opened, thrombosis of the vessels will occur and inflammatory exudate will increase. As the bone is a 'rigid confined space' (sic), the accumulating exudate

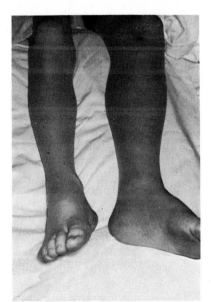

Figure 2.11. The appearance of the limb in acute osteomyelitis of the left tibia in a boy aged 8 years

will cause further vascular occlusions due to rise in pressure. Harris goes on to say, 'By the second or third day, pus has formed, the periosteum is raised over a variable extent and the vascular supply has become compromised: the pus is under considerable pressure and if this is not relieved, thrombosis of vessels may occur, leading inevitably to some degree of bone necrosis.' Thus, if early drainage is, in fact, going to lessen or prevent bone changes, as he repeatedly says, then the surgeon must strike during the interval between the raising of the periosteum by pus and cutting off of the blood supply to the cortex. This is a narrow interval and probably does not exist in practice.

Operations have been performed in 75 children in this series and pus was not encountered under pressure. There was no spurting of pus when the periosteum was incised yet pressure would be essential to the validity of Harris' concept.

Cullen and Glass (1955) found a higher proportion of complications among their cases of acute osteomyelitis who were treated by early operation.

In the earlier years, we treated 2 children by early operation, i.e. within 2 days of onset of severe symptoms and signs and before any radiological change developed.

In 1961, a critically ill boy aged $5\frac{1}{2}$ years was admitted. There was a history of pain in the right upper arm and shoulder for the previous 2 days. He had intense swelling from the right side of the base of the neck down over the clavicle to the elbow (*Figure 2.12*). His temperature was 39.5°C and his ESR was 40. Intravenous saline was set up and benzylpenicillin added to the infusion. It was thought that osteomyelitis of the clavicle with possibly a deep abscess was causing venous obstruction of the arm. A 3-inch incision was made into the infraclavicular foss. No abnormality was found. The wound was closed. The next day, he was no better. It was then thought that the maximum tenderness was at the lower end of the humerus medially and consequently a second exploration was done, again finding oedematous soft tissue but no pus. Sixteen days later, radiographs showed osteomyelitis of the shaft of the humerus. The infection was due to *Staph. aureus* resistant to benzylpenicillin, but sensitive to chloramphenicol. It was instructive to see that radiographs at 16 days showed no new bone formation over the site of operation, the purpose of which was to prevent widespread necrosis.

A boy aged 3 years presented with severe pain of 2 days' duration. Radiographs were normal (*Figure 2.13*). It was possible by locating the point of maximum tenderness to be sure that the metaphyseal abscess was in the lower medial humerus. An incision was made. The periosteum was thickened but not elevated. A gutter was cut into the outer humeral shaft and a small quantity of pus welled into the wound. It seemed that if early operation to decompress the abscess had benefit then this child should not show bone destruction. His radiograph at 10 days showed a typical appearance of osteomyelitis in this site. This became chronic and was still discharging 4 months later. The end result was satisfactory.

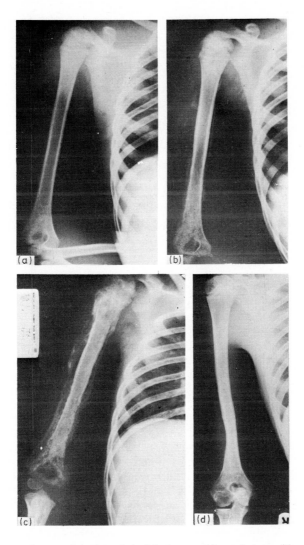

Figure 2.12. Osteomyelitis of the shaft of the humerus (a) on admission; (b) at 16 days; (c) at 24 days; (d) after 9 years

(By courtesy *J. Bone Jt Surg.*, 1970)

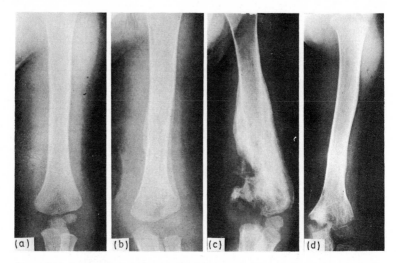

Figure 2.13. Lower humeral osteomyelitis (a) at onset; (b) at 10 days; (c) at 4 months with chronic disease; and finally (d) 3 years later. A failure of primary treatment

Conclusions

These examples show that the site of infection can be difficult to determine, and that even if the exact site is known, no benefit of early operation accrues.

The literature does not contain a series of cases where early operation has given minimal bone destruction.

Some writers (Harris, 1962) have tried to define 'early' in terms of hours since the first symptom. These features are subjective; pathology is objective. A child 48 hours after the first symptoms may have an early lesion or a late one in pathological terms. Fewer than 25 per cent of children in this series had a history of less than 48 hours (*see* Table 2.1). A long history may mean mismanagement and therefore advanced disease, but it may mean an infection of low virulence. Table 2.1, relating failure to length of history, shows that failures are evenly distributed, and not confined to late cases.

The amount of 'necrosis' that results in this disease depends upon the advancement of the lesion at the time when effective antibiotic treatment begins. The length of history is an inaccurate indication of this progress. Necrosis depends on no other factor.

The role of surgery is to evacuate an abscess. It confers no other benefit on the bone or on the child.

In Britain nowadays, it is possible using effective antibiotics to keep the failure rate as low as 10 per cent, surgery being used only for evacuation of any abscess that may form. The advocates of early surgery have not produced clinical or statistical evidence to support their claims. They admit that early operation sometimes does not produce pus but claim that 'oedema' is released and this is beneficial.

Observation suggests that once pus is under the periosteum the medullary cavity is already decompressed. Further evidence for this natural decompression is the failure to find intramedullary pus under pressure.

Rest and antibiotics will cause the inflammation to localize and relieve the intense pain of this disease. When this localization occurs the inflammatory oedema subsides or an area of fluctuation develops in the centre of the lesion. Operation at this time, and no earlier, is the course to take.

THE F.A.T. CATECHISM

All clinicians having experience of treating bacterial infections will have met the problem of lack of clinical response to the agents prescribed. McAllister (1975) has developed a 'Failed Antibiotic Therapy' (F.A.T.) catechism in an attempt to concentrate the clinician's mind on the likely cause. The questions he should ask are suggested by:

(1) Wrong organism, i.e. a wrong guess or a laboratory mistake.
(2) Wrong antibiotic—out-of-date information.
(3) Inappropriate case—wrong diagnosis.
(4) Inadequate dosage.
(5) Antibiotic not getting at the causative bacteria—? need for surgery.
(6) Wrong route of administration.
(7) Inadequate duration.
(8) Development of resistance.
(9) Antibiotic antagonism.
(10) Poor supportive therapy.

We have met all these causes at one time or another and their significance has been discussed in this text. Cause 5 has been the most frequent recently whereas Causes 2, 4 and 8 plagued us in earlier years.

ACUTE OSTEOMYELITIS IN INFANTS

A combination of active early treatment with long-term follow-up of those who presented too late has led to a less gloomy view of this disease than hitherto. Though the principles of treatment remain the same at any age there are differences in presentation. Fourteen children have been studied.

Diagnosis

At the time of diagnosis radiographs always reveal the nature and site of the disease in infants. Their clinical state is not as grave as might be suggested by the radiographic changes. They all have abscesses which are not as hot or tender as in older children. The pathognomonic physical signs are fullness around a joint and pseudoparalysis. These features can be mistaken for local injury or viral infection of the lower motor neurone. Any baby having these two physical signs should be considered to have an acute bone or joint infection until proved otherwise. Pyrexia, failure to thrive and leucocytosis are often not evident until it is too late to save the joint.

Bacteriology and mode of infection

As all 14 infants whose long-term follow-up is here reported had abscesses on admission which were drained the organism was easily identified. There were 13 with benzylpenicillin-resistant Staph. aureus and 1 with H. influenzae.

Recent trends

In 1957 Hurst found that 99 per cent of 106 infants born in hospital carried pathogenic staphylococci on the day they went home. Because of this and other high figures published, the bathing of all neonates in 3 per cent hexachlorophane soon after birth became a routine. The effect of this policy has been striking and suggests a likely decrease in neonatal osteomyelitis secondary to colonization in hospital. McAllister (1975) has shown that even now large numbers of pathogenic organisms can be grown from infants within 1 hour of birth. The incidence of Staph. aureus was 2.6 per cent from infants' umbilical stumps at 2 days old and 4 per cent from their noses on the 7th day. If non-pathogens are disregarded the Gram-negative organisms grown from all sites outnumber the Gram-positive.

Although we are not certain of the mode of infection in any of the 8 infants under 1 month of age with acute osteomyelitis that we have treated in the last 2 years the organism has been:

Staph. aureus (resistant to benzylpenicillin)	4
Strep. pneumoniae	1*
H. influenzae	1
Ps. aeruginosa	1
Staph. albus	1

*This baby with Strep. pneumoniae aged 3 weeks was admitted with a swelling of the left elbow and pseudoparalysis. She was given fusidic acid and erythromycin

The follow-up study

Whilst acute osteomyelitis with or without pyogenic arthritis is serious and often crippling there have been examples of surprising healing and reconstruction resulting more from normal processes than the clinician's efforts.

Figure 2.14a is a radiograph of the knee of a baby presenting with a large joint swelling alleged to have been present only 2 days; 60 ml of pus were evacuated from the joint. *Figure 2.14b* shows the same knee 4 years later. The resistance of the epiphyseal growth plate to destruction shown has been seen in 3 other infants' knees rendering the end result much better than could be expected.

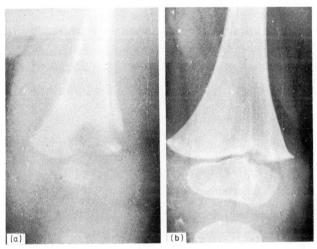

Figure 2.14. (a) Anteroposterior radiograph of an infant's knee. Sixty ml of pus were evacuated. (b) Four years later the knee was normal

Figure 2.15 shows the progression over 8 years of a baby with pyogenic arthritis of the left knee in which both major bones were involved.

Even more advanced destruction with sequestration and sinus formation has with time produced an acceptable result. *Figure 2.16* shows lateral radiographs over 12 years of a neonate infected with benzylpenicillin-resistant *Staph. aureus*. The only operation performed was draining an abscess. Cloxacillin was given for 6 weeks;

---

following aspiration. She remained unwell and on the 6th day developed signs of meningitis. A second elbow aspiration and a cerebrospinal fluid (CSF) tap cultured *Strep. pneumoniae* which settled on intrathecal benzylpenicillin. Thus if this baby had never come near a teaching hospital and had been given benzylpenicillin for her elbow infection by someone not steeped in modern chemotherapy she would have been better served!

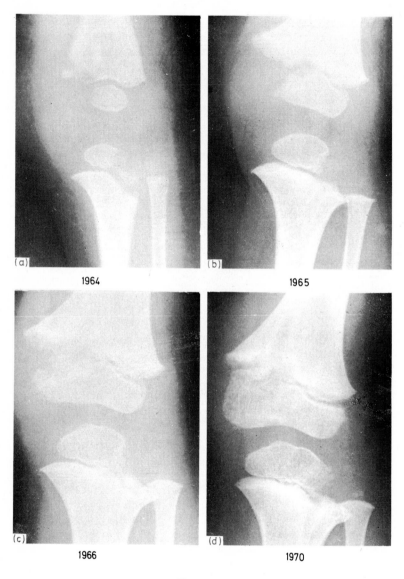

1964   1965

1966   1970

Figure 2.15

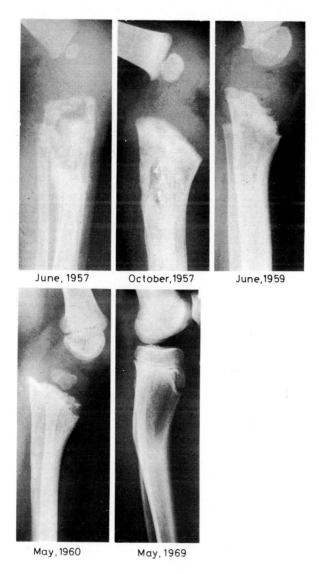

June, 1957 October, 1957 June, 1959

May, 1960 May, 1969

Figure 2.16. The progression in 12 years of upper tibial neonatal osteomyelitis. Note absorption of the sequestrum, a feature only seen in infants

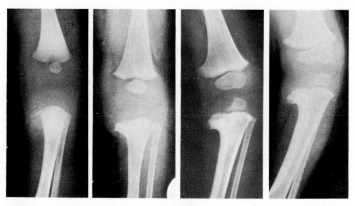

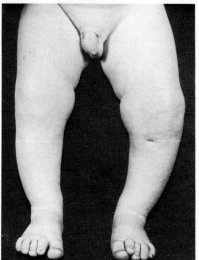

Figure 2.17. The progression over 12 years of an osteomyelitic lesion of the medial tibial condyle of a male infant. The first radiograph was taken at age 1 month, the second radiograph and the clinical photograph were taken at age 10 months and subsequent radiographs show the position at approximately 2-year intervals. The medial tibial condyle, thought to be destroyed, re-forms and the varus improves

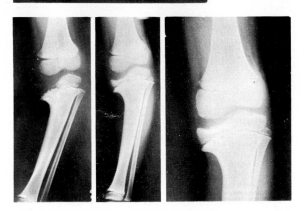

the sequestrum absorbed within 4 months; then 2 years after sterilization an upper tibial epiphysis began to ossify and produced a normal tibial head. There is, in addition to the healing, a tendency towards angular improvement.

Figure 2.17 shows the result over 12 years in a baby with pyogenic arthritis secondary to osteomyelitis of the medial tibial condyle. The second radiograph and the clinical photograph were taken when standing began at age 10 months. Severe bow leg looked inevitable but after a phase of worsening there was progressive improvement leading to minimal deformity.

The shoulders have shown only 2 out of 4 good results. In 2 children a varus deformity had persisted. This is because of epiphyseal slip caused by the infection.

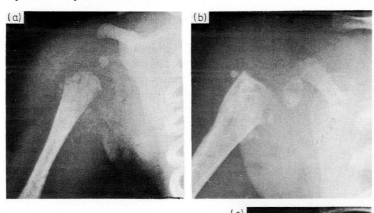

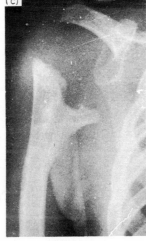

Figure 2.18. A poor result of upper humeral osteomyelitis in an infant due to epiphyseal slip. Progression over 5 years

Figure 2.18 shows pyogenic arthritis of the shoulder in a baby aged 2 weeks (*a*), the position after healing (*b*) and the result 5 years later (*c*).

Humerus varus was also seen in a slightly older infant following acute osteomyelitis due to *Staph. aureus* and again there has been a pathological epiphyseal separation (*Figure 2.19*). The last radiograph shows the 5-year result.

Even with very extensive destruction the remodelling that follows sterilization of the lesion can produce a normal joint provided epiphyseal separation does not occur.

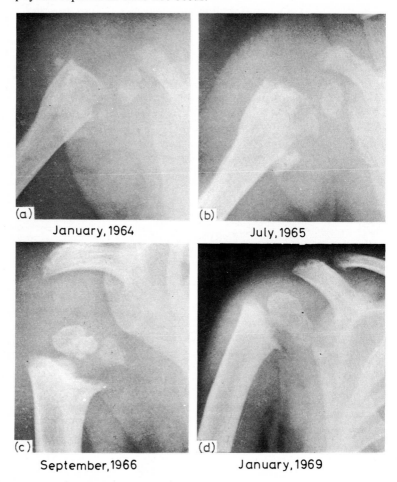

(a) January, 1964   (b) July, 1965

(c) September, 1966   (d) January, 1969

Figure 2.19. The progress over 5 years in a baby aged 6 months at onset of infection

Figure 2.20 shows the 7-year result of a baby who at age 1 month was admitted to the medical side with a pseudoparalysis thought to be due to Erb's palsy. The organism was *H. influenzae.*

Ankylosis was not seen in any of these infants in spite of the fact that in each one the joints contained pus.

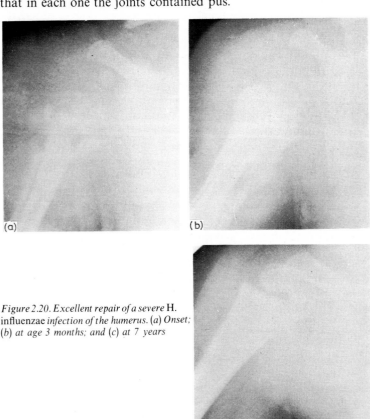

Figure 2.20. Excellent repair of a severe H. influenzae *infection of the humerus.* (a) *Onset;* (b) *at age 3 months; and* (c) *at 7 years*

The hip

Perhaps the greatest interest is taken in the hip because dislocation tends to follow the pyogenic arthritis which is itself secondary to osteomyelitis of the femoral neck. Tom Smith in 1874 described pyogenic arthritis of infancy and pointed out that, if not fatal, recovery occurred without leaving persistent sinuses or late complications. From 13 post-mortem studies he showed that pus entered the joint from rupture of an osteomyelitic abscess. His name is attached to the hip affliction because he had seen 3 pathological dislocations among 8 children who survived.

This dislocation can be very rapid and once established is irreducible. Its avoidance demands the early diagnosis and correct management of the arthritis. In none of the 8 cases here reported, however, was the diagnosis made until after the dislocation had occurred. Distension of the joint, a flexion deformity and pseudoparalysis are the

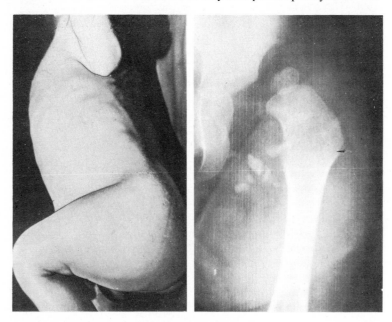

Figure 2.21. The classic signs of suppurative arthritis of the left hip in the infant and the radiographic appearance

diagnostic features (*Figure 2.21*). The joint should immediately be opened through a posterior muscle-splinting incision, the abscess evacuated, the hip reduced and the wound closed holding the thigh in a position of reduction. Appropriate antibiotics are, as usual, essential.

Although we have always acted later than desirable the results have been satisfying.

Figure 2.22 shows suppurative dislocation of the right hip of a baby aged 3 weeks due to septicaemic spread from an umbilical stump.

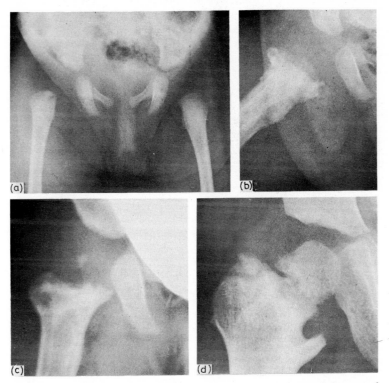

Figure 2.22. The progress over 7 years of suppurative arthritis of the right hip treated by open drainage and reduction of the dislocation. Radiographs (a) at onset; (b) at 2 months; (c) at 1 year; and (d) at 7 years

The joint was opened and drained and then immobilized in abduction. Later radiographs showed the true extent of the femoral disease. The prognosis was guarded because it was assumed that the femoral head had been destroyed.

However, over the next 7 years the joint returned to normal and the only permanent defect was a shortened irregular femoral neck.

If the primary focus is acetabular, remodelling does not occur. *Figure 2.23* shows dislocation of the joint of a boy in whom this was the case. Sixty ml of staphylococcal pus were extracted from the joint, reduction achieved and antibiotics continued for 6 weeks. The last figure shows the same hip 10 years later. The joint is stable but the limb is 1 inch short and the capital epiphysis has not formed.

An alarming event interrupted the management of another infant with suppurative arthritis of the hip. The hip was opened at 3 weeks old. After evacuation of the abscess the frog position was adjudged

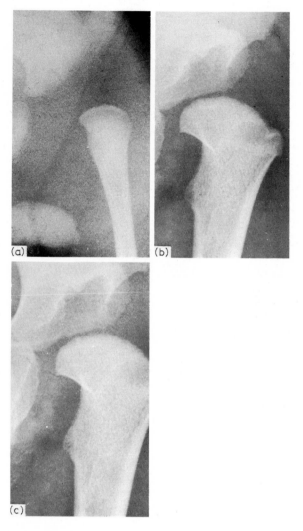

Figure 2.23. The progression over 10 years in a boy whose septic arthritis was secondary to acetabular disease. Remodelling has not occurred

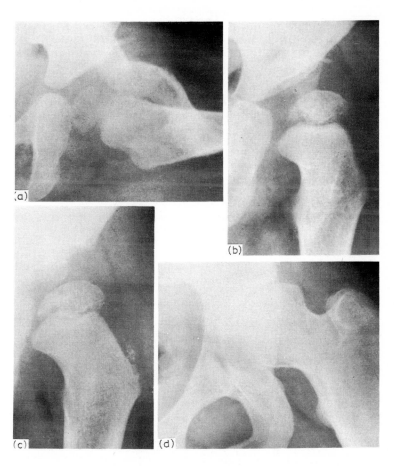

Figure 2.24. Bony ankylosis of the hip following drainage of suppurative arthritis of infancy and immobilization in the frog position (a). Radiographs show progress at 1 year (b); at 3 years (c); and at 17 years (d)

the best way of holding the reduction achieved. The plaster was removed after 3 months and the hip was ankylosed. Radiographs
revealed an extracapsular mature bar of bone totally fixing the hip
(*Figure 2.24*). It was decided to explore the hip from the front and
remove this bar of bone before encouraging movements. One year
later the hip looked unstable but 17 years later the hip was normal.
The patient was playing hockey for the school team.

Two cases of suppurative arthritis of infancy had dislocation which
persisted. In both an attempted open reduction failed totally.

PERMANENT DEFORMITY

Figure 2.25 shows the lateral aspect of the femur in a girl aged 12
involved with chronic osteomyelitis. The sequestrum was removed

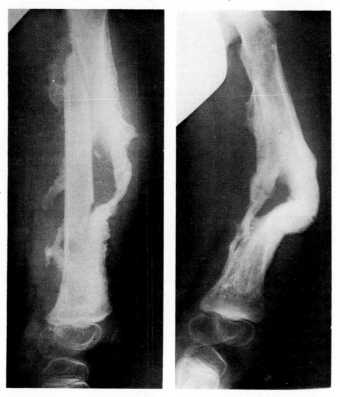

*Figure 2.25. Sequestrectomy performed too early. Six months after operation shortening
was noticed which did not improve*

along with all infected tissue. Six months later shortening and anterior femoral bowing had occurred. It would have been wiser to delay the sequestrectomy until a stronger involucrum had formed.

Most permanent deformities in this disease are due to the only complication mentioned, in the first paragraph of this chapter (*see* page 15), which is untreatable, i.e. epiphyseal growth plate damage.

Figure 2.26 is a radiograph of the almost useless forearm of a lady aged 45 years who described 7 operations and prolonged stays in hospital between the ages of 2 and 7 years.

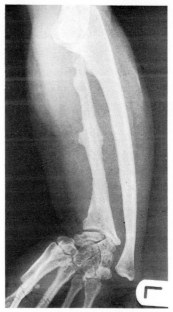
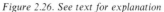
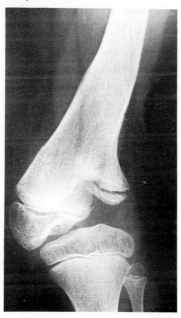

Figure 2.26. See text for explanation   *Figure 2.27. See text for explanation*

Figure 2.27 is a radiograph of the knee of a child aged 11 years whose infantile infection of the lateral femoral condyle did not behave as the infant's depicted in *Figure 2.14a* (*see* page 41). There is shortening, instability and valgus requiring a caliper and raised shoe while awaiting arthrodesis.

A girl aged 9 years was too unusual to be omitted. She presented with feet pointing in different directions (*Figure 2.28a*), which, when she was lying down, were grotesque (*Figure 2.28b*). This deformity was due to pathological separation of the upper tibial epiphyseal plate, allowing the lower leg to externally rotate 180 degrees. By a two-stage osteotomy it was possible to correct the deformity (*Figure 2.28c*).

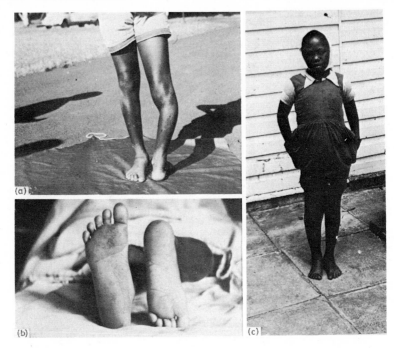

Figure 2.28. The correction of a 180 degree angular deformity by osteotomy

SUBACUTE OSTEOMYELITIS

Clinical features

The complaint is of aching pain, swelling and disability of some months' duration. There is often pain at night. The affected metaphysis is slightly enlarged giving the impression that the bone is thicker than normal at that site. There is no general upset and no history of previous acute infection. Temperature and sedimentation rate are normal or slightly raised. The condition has been well described by King and Mayo (1969).

Radiological features

Radiographs show a well-demarcated metaphyseal lesion without periosteal reaction and without surrounding sclerosis. These changes are present on the child's first attendance at hospital. *Figure 2.29* and *2.30* are typical examples.

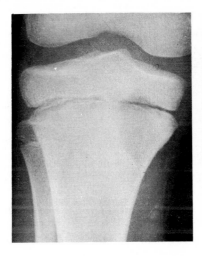 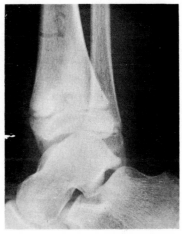

Figure 2.29. Subacute osteomyelitis of the tibia

Figure 2.30. Subacute osteomyelitis of the lower tibia

Differential diagnosis

Congenital fibrous defect, benign neoplasm and eosinophil granuloma can all give similar clinical and radiological features.

Prevalence

In the 10 years of this study of 300 children with clinical acute osteomyelitis in 151 of whom proof was obtained, 27 presented with subacute osteomyelitis. Thus the prevalence of subacute compared to proven acute infections is 1 to 6.

Site

Sixteen lesions were situated in the upper tibial metaphysis and the other 11 in the metaphyses elsewhere including one in the spinous process of the third lumbar vertebra.

Treatment

All these lesions were opened and evacuated for diagnostic and therapeutic purposes. The organisms cultured were:

Staph. *aureus* sensitive to benzylpenicillin   8
Staph. *aureus* resistant to benzylpenicillin   12
Other   7
                                                      ——
                                                      27

After evacuation and 21 days' effective antibiotics the lesions healed in a fashion similar to that described previously for infected metaphyseal lesions in children (*see* page 25).

Conclusions

The length of history, the quiet presentation and the presence of radiographic changes at the start distinguish this lesion from acute osteomyelitis. The absence of sclerosis on radiographs distinguishes it from Brodie's abscess. The classification of this lesion into six types (King and Mayo, 1969) is unduly elaborate. The diagnostic criteria are older children, longer history, less acute physical signs, little radiological sclerosis and no periosteal reaction.

BRODIE'S ABSCESS

In 1832, Benjamin Brodie described 3 young men who came under his care, complaining of swelling and intermittent severe pain over the tibia for between 10 and 18 years. The characteristics common to all were 'adherence of the integument to the underlying bone' and, at operation '*a central cavity the size of a walnut containing dark-coloured pus surrounded by white dense bone*'. The cavity was opened by using a trephine through a cruciate incision. A concoction of sarsaparilla had been ineffective. The first patient died, aged 24, of what sounds like meningitis secondary to septicaemia following amputation. Brodie describes the white dense bone as 'not less than one-third of an inch thick and manifestly the result of inflammation of the periosteum at some former period'.

The length of history in his 3 male patients was 12 years, 10 years and 18 years. Although it was considered that these lesions were the result of previous inflammation, there is no concrete evidence of this. None of the 3 described acute osteomyelitis in early childhood and none showed scars or sinuses which suggested that diagnosis.

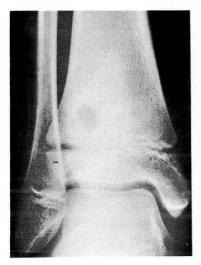 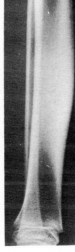 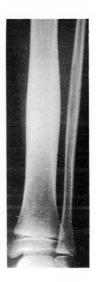

Figure 2.31. Anteroposterior radiograph of classic Brodie's abscess in a boy aged 9 years with a 9-month history

Figure 2.32. Lateral and anteroposterior radiographs of the tibia of a girl aged 6 years who experienced pain in the leg intermittently for 1 year

It is clear that whatever the cause of these lesions, the essential criteria for diagnosis are the long history and the surrounding sclerosis.

In the period of 10 years spent studying pyogenic infections of bone in children, only 2 cases satisfying these criteria have presented. *Figures 2.31* and *2.32* are radiographs showing these 2 lesions.

TABLE 2.2

Relationship of the Three Types of Pyogenic Bone Infection in Children in a 10-year Period at Royal Hospital for Sick Children, Glasgow

Proven acute osteomyelitis	151
Subacute osteomyelitis	27
Brodie's abscess	2

If we confine the term 'Brodie's abscess' to conditions complying with his description, the incidence in children is extremely low. The diagnostic criteria are a long history, night pain and marked surrounding sclerosis on radiographs. Children have not lived long enough to develop the last feature.

REFERENCES

Blockey, N. J. and McAllister, T. A. (1972). *J. Bone Jt Surg.* **54B,** 299
— and Watson, J. T. (1970). *J. Bone Jt Surg.* **52B,** 77
Br. med. J. (1974). Leading article **4,** 65
Brodie, B. (1832). *Med. chir. Trans.* **17,** 239.
Craven, J. L., Pugsley, D. J. and Blowers, R. (1970). *Br. med. J.* **3,** 201
Cullen, C. H. and Glass, A. (1955). *J. Bone Jt Surg.* **37B,** 722
Deodhar, S. D., Russel, F., Carson Dick, W., Nuki, G. and Buchanan, W. W. *Scand. J. Rheum.* **1,** 33
Green, J. H. (1967). *Br. med. J.* **2,** 144
Harris, N. H. (1962). *Br. med. J.* **1,** 1437
Hurst, V. (1957). *H. Hyg., Camb.* **55,** 299
Jackson, G. G. and Arcieri, G. (1971). *J. infect. Dis.* **124,** 130
Jensen, K. and Lassen, H. C. A. (1969). *Q. Jl Med.* **149,** 91
Jones, J. (1974). Personal communication
King, D. M. and Mayo, K. M. (1969). *J. Bone Jt Surg.* **41B,** 458
Lack, C. H. and Towers, A. C. (1962). *Br. med. J.* **2,** 1227
Larsen, R. M. (1934). *Ann. Surg.* **108,** 127
McAllister, T. A. (1975). *Scott. med. J.* (In press)
Maudsley, R. H. and Taylor, A. R. (1970). *J. Bone Jt Surg.* **52B,** 58
Ridley, M., Lynn, R., Barrie, D. and Stead, K. C. (1970). *Lancet* **1,** 230
Rowling, D. E. (1969). *J. Bone Jt Surg.* **41B,** 681
Schandling, B. (1960). *S. Afr. med. J.* **34,** 520
Smith, I. M. (1971). *Post-grad. med. J.* February supplement, p. 78
Spink, W. W. (1956). *Ann. N.Y. Acad. Sci.* **65,** 175
Trueta, J. (1957). *J. Bone Jt Surg.* **39B,** 358
Walker, S. H. (1973). *Clin. Pediat.* **12,** 98

3 The Swollen Knee

The knee is the joint most commonly found to be involved in children's orthopaedics. Whilst some conditions are easily recognized and simply treated others demand specialized knowledge often thought to be outside an orthopaedic surgeon's field. For the benefit of those not working closely with clinicians of other disciplines some of these ailments are dealt with here.

We have to consider the differential diagnosis and management of swelling of the knee joint itself. Pre-patellar bursitis and traumatic synovitis have not been included as they present no problem.

The clinical picture is that of a child with a tense swelling of one knee who is seen either in the casualty or outpatient department (*Figure 3.1*).

FRACTURES

The commonest fracture involving the knee joint of children is avulsion of the tibial table. Such patients can present with a warm, swollen, slightly flexed knee without a definite history of hyperflexion or hyper-rotation. The anteroposterior radiograph can look normal in such cases but the lateral view will reveal the avulsed table. This is hinged posteriorly and can easily be missed. Under general anaesthesia the joint should be aspirated and then placed into full extension and a lateral radiograph taken. If the fragment has not been pushed back by the femur the joint should be opened, blood clot removed from the always large tibial crater and the tibial spines sutured back to their bed. A groin-to-ankle plaster with the knee in full extension for 4 weeks gives good results. Although plaster in full extension is abhorred by some (Sharrard, 1971) we have seen no complications from its use.

HAEMARTHROSIS

Traumatic haemarthrosis without fracture should also be managed by aspiration under anaesthesia.

The swollen knee in the boy with haemophilia or Christmas disease presents no difficulty in diagnosis. Haemarthroses in these conditions rarely present under age 2 years. In haemophilia, it is the anti-haemophilic globulin, Factor VIII, which is deficient and the patient liable to spontaneous haemarthrosis is the child with about 1 per cent or less of the normal Factor VIII level. Those with a level of 2 per cent or more tend to present with haemarthroses or soft-tissue haematomata only after trauma. They are treated with immediate replacement therapy followed by bedrest traction and quadriceps drill after the swelling recedes. Acute haemarthrosis in coagulation disorders should be aspirated if the swelling is both tense and painful. Repeated conservative management has in our experience led to erosion of articular cartilage and permanent anyklosis in some older children. Our policy with severe haemarthrosis of the knee in haemophilia is now as follows: cryoprecipitate is used in preference to fresh-frozen plasma because its dose can be increased two- or fourfold without embarrassment to the circulation. Two units per 10 kg bodyweight are rapidly injected iv (raising the Factor VIII level by about 20 per cent). Aspiration of the joint is carried out under strict aseptic precautions—the dose of cryoprecipitate is then repeated every 12 hours for 48 hours giving during this period a Factor VIII level of about 30 per cent of normal. This level will then fall at a rate of half for every 12 hours and may thus not reach unsafe levels again for a further 48 hours. If fresh-frozen plasma is used the dose recommended is 15 ml/kg bodyweight infused over half to one hour and again repeated every 12 hours for 48 hours. This regime is used in Christmas disease (Factor IX deficiency) where cryoprecipitate would be of no value. The destruction of Factor IX being slower than that of Factor VIII, daily rather than 12-hourly doses are necessary. Major surgery requires that the Factor VIII level never falls below 30 per cent (or Factor IX below 15 per cent) at any time during the 10 days until wound healing is secure. These levels cannot be maintained by the use of fresh-frozen plasma because of hypervolaemia. In haemophilia cryoprecipitate or the more recently available human Factor VIII concentrates (e.g. Hemofil, Hyland) are satisfactory; in Christmas disease Factor IX concentrate (e.g. Konyne, Cutter) is necessary. Similar concentrates are now becoming available through the Blood Transfusion Service in Britain. Animal (bovine or porcine) Factor VIII would only be used if a human concentrate was unavailable or if the patient had circulating inhibitors to Factor VIII.

If anaemia is present it should be corrected by the slow infusion of packed red cells after appropriate replacement therapy. 'Fresh' whole blood is not indicated.

Prompt relief of tension and cessation of bleeding into the knee has greatly improved the lot of the severe haemophiliac. Quadriceps drill can be begun early and weight-bearing with caliper or splint continued. These patients can now expect a long life. Although their defects do not change each bleed is less damaging with modern management and their avoidance of trauma contributes to longevity. Unfortunately progressive arthropathy is still seen in older patients whose earlier bleeds were managed in a previous therapeutic era.

'Early warning' treatment at home is now being tested. A responsible relative gives an iv injection at the first sign of a haemarthrosis. This technique requires the patient to have good veins and the household to possess a deep freeze to store the cryoprecipitate at $-20°C$. It is likely to mean fewer days off school and earlier coagulation correction than the usual journey to hospital but there are dangers of increased consumption, of allergic reactions and of sepsis. Factor VIII concentrate Hemofil does not require a deep freeze for safekeeping, but its cost is high. For the very severely affected patient intermittent prophylactic replacement therapy is used; 20 units/kg of Factor VIII every 48 hours has been shown to keep the level about 1 per cent, i.e. above the level producing spontaneous haemorrhage. In Christmas disease the longer half-life of Factor IX allows effective prophylaxis from 10 units/kg twice weekly (Willoughby, 1974).

JUVENILE RHEUMATOID ARTHRITIS (JRA)

When this generalized disease begins as a monarthritis difficulties of diagnosis arise. The knee is warm, tightly swollen, flexed, painful and shows considerable thigh muscle wasting (*Figure 3.1*). The diagnosis is suggested by the physical signs, a raised ESR and radiological evidence of epiphyseal enlargement, of osteoporosis without specific bone erosion and by slight increase in length of the limb—these findings are invariable if the joint disease has been present for 3 months or more. Radiographs of the chest and a strict intradermal Mantoux test 1 in 1000 tend to distinguish the cooler joint of tuberculous arthritis. If no other joint is involved and no stigmata of juvenile rheumatoid arthritis are present elsewhere the diagnosis cannot be substantiated without open biopsy examination. Upon diagnosis we advise a period of bedrest on a Thomas splint with below-knee extensions whilst giving acetylsalicyclic acid 4-hourly sufficent to hold the blood salicylate level at 20–30 mg/100 ml for 6 weeks. This is followed by physiotherapy and night splintage to retain extension and quadriceps power.

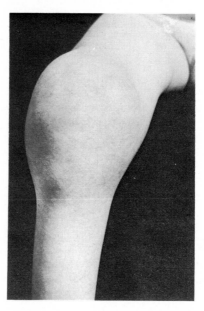

Figure 3.1. The swollen knee. Clinical features in a boy aged 4 years with rheumatoid arthritis

Biopsy is necessary for proof (Ansell and Bywaters, 1959). The open operation is preferred. Rheumatoid synovium is pink or purple whereas tuberculous synovium is grey and the fluid contains flecks. The histological tissue reaction is seldom diagnostic but must be studied with other evidence before rheumatoid arthritis is confirmed. The pathologist can exclude other more serious diseases. We have 5 cases presenting as monarthritis with features similar to those who later fell into the category of JRA in whom the suggestive histological tissue reaction had other causes. One child had a small fragment of chicken bone in the knee and in a second child culture of the synovium grew *E. coli*, the inflammatory process settling after appropriate antibiotics (*Figure 3.2*).

Thus the diagnosis of rheumatoid arthritis is made too often in cases of children with monarthritis. When the diagnosis is confirmed, too gloomy a view is often taken of the outcome. In the 28 years 1942–70 100 children were admitted to the Royal Hospital for Sick Children, Glasgow, and have recently been extensively studied (Goel and Shanks, 1974). The diagnostic criteria of Ansell and Bywaters (1959) were used. Only 9 of these presented as monarthritis, 7 with

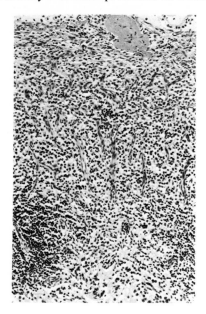

Figure 3.2. Histology (× 50) demonstrating difficulty in interpretation. The synovial surface is at the top where polymorphs are seen. Bottom left is a lymphoid follicle. There are lymphocytes and plasma cells in the underlying layers of the synovium. These features made rheumatoid arthritis impossible to exclude. (This synovial biopsy was taken from a boy aged 12 years with an E. coli synovitis of 7 days' duration, warm joint and ESR 84 mm in one hour)

involvement of the knee joint, 1 with a swollen ankle and 1 with a wrist synovitis. These 9 children have been followed up for from $1\frac{1}{2}$ to 9 years. In 3 of them only did other joints become involved. One child presenting with right knee joint swelling gradually developed over the next 3 years swellings of the left knee and of the right ankle. A second child again presenting with right knee swelling developed within 18 months swellings of the left knee. The third child presented with synovitis of the left ankle and within the first 6 weeks developed arthritis in both knees. No other joint changes were seen in the subsequent 9 years. Eight of the 9 children whose rheumatoid disease presented as monarthritis had a negative Rose Waaler test both at the time of onset and at follow-up. The 1 child whose Rose Waaler test was positive (titre of 1 in 64 or more) presented as a right knee swelling and was the only one whose knee was not operated on for biopsy examination. The Rose Waaler test was negative 8 years later. At follow-up all these 9 had quiescent disease. Eight had no limitation of function and 1 had two stiff knees giving moderate restriction of activity. From the 100 children with rheumatoid arthritis, 16 were found to be severely disabled at follow-up but 15 of these had an onset of disease either with generalized polyarthritis or with acute development of generalized systemic manifestations. A positive family history of rheumatoid arthritis was found in close relatives from 12 of the 100 patients (52 girls and 48 boys). The 9 monarticular presentations, our main concern, occurred in 6 girls and 3 boys of ages 9 months to $10\frac{1}{2}$ years. In 6, all proved by biopsy, the disease remained confined to one joint. Thus in an 18-year period a large children's hospital can expect 9 of the many children presenting with a solitary swollen major joint to have rheumatoid arthritis. The Rose Waaler is likely to be negative, spread to more than two other joints will not occur and serious permanent disability is most unlikely.

This experience is similar to that of Bywaters and Ansell (1965). They studied 316 cases of Still's disease in children in 15 years and 33 of these cases presented as monarthritis (i.e. the child had pain and swelling without any other joint becoming involved for 3 months.) In 23 of them the knee joint was involved. In 14 of the 33 beginning as monarthritis, the disease remained confined to one joint (mean follow-up 6.5 years). In 7 it progressed to 1 or 2 other joints and in 12 there occurred more generalized involvement. Fifteen of the 19 getting further joint involvement did so within the first year. The Rose Waaler test was positive in only 1 of the 33 cases (in only 1 of our patients was the Rose Waaler test positive, too) but of the 28 biopsies performed features typical or suggestive of rheumatoid arthritis were seen. As in our patients there was no correlation between the original biopsy findings and the ultimate course of the disease.

ACUTE RHEUMATISM

Again the knee is commonly involved. The child, usually aged 7 years or more, is flushed, toxic and ill. The joint is tender on all aspects, there is a marked synovial effusion which feels hot. The joint is held slightly flexed and a small range of movement only is permitted.

There is often a history of sore throat some days previously and no history of injury. A complete examination is necessary as the local picture is similar to that of haemarthrosis or acute pyogenic infection. To substantiate a diagnosis of acute rheumatism when a single joint is involved one must have some of the following features: cardiomegaly or at least tachycardia with a lengthened PR interval on the ECG; erythema marginatum; visible and/or palpable spots lying subcutaneously (the extensor aspects of the elbows or the occipital region of the scalp are typical sites for these Aschoff nodules); a raised temperature, raised ESR and an ASO titre over 1000 units/ml.

In our experience another joint often becomes acutely involved within 2 to 4 days of onset often with spontaneous improvement of the first joint involved, hence the classic description of 'fleeting and flitting arthritis'. If the diagnosis is in doubt aspiration is advisable— the fluid is thin, yellowish and present in large quantities (in one instance, 80 ml from the knee of a child aged 8 years). It contains polymorphs and no organisms. These features are unlike those of joints acutely infected with pyogenic organisms. If aspiration is not performed a short period of rest in bed and the oral administration of salicylate 4 g/day increasing if necessary until signs of mild salicylism (deafness, tinnitus) develop, should be given. Non-resolution of an acutely inflamed joint within 24 hours of beginning this treatment would be strongly against a diagnosis of acute rheumatism. This diagnosis should only be reached after careful consideration—it should not be used for any painful swollen joint not due to trauma whose synovial fluid is sterile. The diagnosis demands a twice daily dose of oral penicillin for perhaps 15 years and, of course, carries implications for future life insurance.

ACUTE PYOGENIC INFECTIONS

Children admitted with acute pyogenic arthritis are usually aged between 1 and 5 years. The joint is hot, swollen and tender. It is not easy in this age group to distinguish the tenderness of acute osteomyelitis from that of arthritis in the younger end of this age group and the former condition can often produce a sympathetic effusion. In pyogenic arthritis there is inhibition of active joint movement— pseudoparalysis—and visible enlargement of all aspects of the joint. The temperature, ESR and white cell count are raised and radiographic evidence of enlargement of soft tissues is seen. Blood culture should be performed and the management should be that for acute osteomyelitis with rest, splintage and antibiotics. The causative bacteria are in our experience the same as those for osteomyelitis except that pyogenic arthritis at under age 2 years, particularly if the ankle is involved, has been due to *H. influenzae* far more often than the 2.5 per cent incidence of this pathogen in acute osteomyelitis in children. The commonest organism is still *Staph. aureus*, however. If there is tension and pain at rest aspiration is performed under general anaesthetic. The fluid is cloudy and present in small amounts. It should be injected into blood culture bottles for aerobic and anaerobic culture. Ampicillin and cloxacillin are given for infections at age 2 years or under and fucidin and erythromycin for other infections. I have not been convinced that either repeated aspirations or aspiration followed by intra-articular injections of antibiotics offer an advantage over the management described. Usually the response to treatment is quick and after 10 days if there is no bone infection, movements can be encouraged. Failure so to respond may be due to an unusual infection. A boy aged 12 years developed a pyogenic arthritis of the ankle. Fucidin and erythromycin were given. Ten days later the swelling was more severe with intense osteoporosis. A biopsy was performed and at the same time the synovium and its fluid were cultured. *E. coli* was grown. The histological reaction (*Figure 3.2*) showed features of synovitis with round cell aggregates somewhat suggestive of rheumatoid arthritis. The condition settled completely following a course of ampicillin and rest. Histological tissue reactions of biopsy specimens are often non-specific.

There remain some knee joint swellings in which no diagnosis can be made. The problem can be rendered more difficult by injudicious explorations, arthrography, biopsy or injections.

Observations over a period of time have often helped. Three weeks on a back splint for idiopathic cool effusions, and for warmer knees antibiotics plus bedrest on a Thomas splint with below-knee skin extensions will often allow the diagnosis to declare itself. Two of the worst knees seen in the last 10 years have warned us of the pitfalls of too enthusiastic diagnosis. One was a boy aged 5 years whose swollen right knee was submitted to biopsy and became infected and the second was a girl whose infected knee was injected with chloramphenicol.

Biopsy should be performed if there is a real possibility of tuberculous arthritis. The non-specificity of the synovial reaction to injury or infection is such as to render biopsy of limited value in proving the presence of rheumatoid and allied disorders.

TUBERCULOUS ARTHRITIS

Tuberculosis of the knee has not disappeared. With 11 280 new notifications in England and Wales in 1970 and 1450 deaths, tuberculosis is second only to influenza in its danger. In towns with high immigrant population the incidence is far above the national average and among this population there is a threefold increase of extrapulmonary lesions, many of which are due to atypical mycobacteria.

What bedevils the scientific treatment of bone and joint infection in children is frequent inability to culture the organism and thus assess its sensitivity. Whilst the case of a 'best guess' choice of antibiotic in pyogenic osteomyelitis has been argued and proved wise, a similar attitude is forced on the clinician in tuberculous infections because of inability to find the infecting mycobacterium. The British child most likely to develop tuberculosis of the knee or any other bone or joint is a contact who did not receive *Calmette-Guérin bacillus (BCG) in infancy* or one in later childhood whose immunity from inoculation in infancy has worn off. The infection is likely to be secondary to a *chest* or very rarely a *bowel infection* and to be a human type contacted from an aged human relative. The joint involved will have a cool, firm swelling with marked muscle wasting. The presence of other joint involvement renders the diagnosis of tuberculous arthritis extremely unlikely. A physical sign known to the older generation of Liverpool postgraduate students and attributed to Alexandrof (reference undetermined) is the difficulty in picking up a pinch of skin from the affected joint. The skin, being tethered deeply, slips away from the examining fingers in a fashion not found in the other causes of chronic joint swelling. Radiographs will show osteoporosis and if a bone lesion is present this will appear indefinite as if a cavity has been drawn in in pencil and then smudged with the finger. The essential investigations of such a swelling would include radiographs of the chest, sedimentation rate, examination of gastric washing and urinary specimen for acid-fast bacilli, Mantoux reaction and open biopsy. This last investigation is likely to reveal a grey, thickened synovium with flecks in the joint fluid. An excised portion should be sent for pathological investigation and another portion for bacteriological examination. Both these specimens will be searched for acid-fast bacilli. The clinician will then have evidence from radiographs, from the Mantoux reaction, from the histologist and from the bacteriologist to add to his clinical examination. If all 4 evidences point to tuberculosis the diagnosis is made. However, tuberculosis in recent years has seldom produced such incontrovertible proof of its presence. Bacteriological proof is either not forthcoming or arrives late on the clinical scene.

Of the other evidences, the most important is seeing the typical histological tissue reaction in excised synovium. A patient aged 12 years with a large, cool knee swelling which on biopsy showed typical tuberculous follicles was reported to have a persistently negative Mantoux reaction 1 in 1000. The joint responded well to antituberculous drugs. Another patient with a chronic ankle swelling which was explored and reported as showing acid- and alcohol-fast bacilli did not have the characteristic synovitis of tuberculosis and was consequently not given drugs. Her swelling settled and the mistake in reporting the bacteriological specimen was later discovered.

To prescribe streptomycin, *p*-aminosalicyclic acid, (PAS) and Isoniazid (INAH) for a child demands certain proof of tuberculosis. They are too dangerous to use without this proof. Unless we can develop better ways of culturing this organism, which are not forthcoming, we have to accept the histological proof. The Mantoux reaction is almost diagnostic if properly performed.

Infections in the immigrant population have caused the increased incidence of new cases of tuberculosis in many towns (Blackburn had 140 new cases in 1970, 3 times the figure for 1960). It is here that the likelihood of atypical infections is greater. We have used with value a differential Mantoux test to try to distinguish these in order to select the chemotherapy more intelligently. The volar surfaces of the forearms are used. Five I.T.U. (0.0001 mg) mammalian tuberculin is injected in 0.1 ml intradermally into the left arm and the same dose of avian tuberculin into the right arm. The reactions are read at 48 hours. Erythema is ignored but the minimum and maximum diameter of induration are measured and the means recorded. Ninety per cent of patients with *M. tuberculosis* infection will have an induration of over 12 mm. A 6–10 mm lesion can only be considered a doubtful result which could be a cross-reaction with atypical infection. On the avian side induration of over 5 mm and also 5 mm greater than the mammalian side suggests an atypical mycobacterial infection. This is not specific for *M. avium* but would indicate the importance of getting the organism in any way possible. A history of contact with fowls or soil-eating habits would make an atypical infection more likely.

A child who has had a successful BCG inoculation in infancy is unlikely to contract tuberculosis in the first 10 years of life. This goes for most Scottish children. In England it is commoner to give BCG at age 12–14 years to those who are Mantoux-negative at that age. In the North American continent BCG inoculation is not routinely used in children.

Confirmation of bone or joint infection thought likely to be by *M. tuberculosis* by evidence of the Mantoux reaction or proved so by staining or culture requires streptomycin, PAS and INAH for 6 months in the first instance unless sensitivity tests suggest otherwise. It has been shown elsewhere (Blockey, 1967) that the type of histological tissue reaction should not alter this basic concept. A lesion with a proliferative tissue reaction should not be treated differently from one showing a caseating process.

If the differential Mantoux reaction and home environment suggest an *M. avium* or other atypical infection it is even more important to find an organism to culture. Repeated biopsy, repeated gastric contents and urinary searches should be carried out as streptomycin, INAH and PAS are not likely to be effective in such an infection and yet the more effective drugs ethambutol and rifamycin have other dangers.

M. tuberculosis (bovine and human) looks identical to the other acid–alcohol-fast, Gram-positive bacilli—*M. avium*, etc.—which may cause infection in man. No distinction can be made for 4–6 weeks when cultural characteristics of the latter render them atypical. It is another 6 weeks before sensitivities can be assayed and thus 3 months elapse from first seeing a bacillus to being in a position to decide accurately the chemotherapy to use. Whilst more cases of genuine *M. avium* infections do occur we have twice seen and cultured this organism from gastric washings and urine from a patient with a joint infection. In both cases we have treated the child with streptomycin, Isoniazid and PAS because in both cases the differential Mantoux test indicated a mammalian infection. The response to treatment was good although resistance to the drugs used of the only mycobacterium cultured was reported. We assumed in these cases that the *M. avium* was not responsible for the orthopaedic lesions.

British policy is now to give BCG vaccination to tuberculin-negative children between the ages 10 and 13 years but some local authorities give BCG to infants.

The tuberculin (Mantoux) test using purified protein derivative (PPD) has largely superseded old tuberculin (OT) as one of the most specific tests in clinical medicine. If an infant is tuberculin-positive he must have an active infection which may not be evident. With increasing age the proportion of tuberculin-positive children rises but nowadays only 4 per cent give a positive tuberculin test at routine school examination (in 1950 it was 50 per cent). The tuberculin test can be negative in children who have or have had tuberculous infections if there is severe malnutrition, or terminal disease. A temporary negative test can be seen in children soon after measles vaccination or during corticosteroid therapy.

The small proportion of children who develop tuberculosis in spite of BCG inoculation contract the disease within a period of 6 weeks before and 6 weeks after vaccination.

Progress of a tuberculous arthritis is monitored by the sedimentation rate, the general well-being of the child and serial radiographic examinations. The decision as to whether to allow movement in a synovial infection thought to be healed can still be difficult. If a second biopsy is performed after say, 6 months,of splintage, and antituberculous drugs, a more informed opinion can be given as to the state of the resolution of infection (*see* Blockey and Laurie, 1963). This operation can be performed through the original biopsy scar and can give information not otherwise obtainable.

APPROXIMATE FREQUENCY OF THE DIAGNOSES DISCUSSED

In 50 recent knee joint swellings in children the diagnosis was:

Haemarthrosis	4
Anaphylactoid purpura	1
Tuberculosis	2
Rheumatoid arthritis	2
Acute rheumatism	3
Septic arthritis (proven)	11
Acute osteomyelitis	4
Intra-articular fractures	2
No definite diagnosis	21
	50

It will be seen that almost half the painful swellings of the child's knee coming to an orthopaedic department will not easily fit into any category. For these, time, rest, splintage and quadriceps drill have been our most effective weapons.

Investigation should be thorough but not over-vigorous.

REFERENCES

Ansell, B. M. and Bywaters, E. G. L. (1959). *Bull. rheum. Dis.* **9,** 189
Bywaters, E. G. L. and Ansell, B. M. (1965). *Ann. rheum. Dis.* **24,** 116
Blockey, N. J. (1967). *E. Afr. med. J.* **44,** 307
— and Lawrie, J. (1963). *Scott. med. J.* **8,** 129
Goel, K. M. and Shanks, R. A. (1974). *Ann. rheum. Dis.* **33,** 25
Sharrard, J. W. J. (1971). *Paediatric Orthopaedics and Fractures.* Oxford; Blackwell
Willoughby, M. J. (1974). Personal communication

4 Congenital Dislocation of the Hip

PROBLEMS IN THE NEONATE

Our attention was drawn by Barlow (1962) and Von Rosen (1962) to the 'clunk' sign of the paediatrician Marino Ortolani (1937) which diagnosed congenital dislocation of the hip (CDH) in the newborn.

In consequence lectures were given, charts produced, pamphlets circulated and ciné films rolled to audiences of obstetricians, midwives, nurses and anyone concerned with delivering babies to show them the simple means whereby the sting could be taken out of this condition. In those days we recognized three states of the infant's hip: the normal, the teratological dislocation (pre-natal; rare and probably better not treated at birth) and the hip which was either dislocated or dislocatable. Finlay, Maudesley and Busfield (1967) found 81 hips in this last group in 60 infants from a total of 14 594 births. Von Rosen found 68 unstable hips among 31 200 newborn infants, and Barlow found 168 dislocated hips and another 186 dislocatable hips among 19 625 newborn infants. These figures refer to findings of examinations by Ortolani's test or Barlow's modifications of it performed at birth. And yet the best estimate of the incidence of true CDH is 0.65 per 1000 live births, put forward by Record and Edwards (1958) who studied children born in Birmingham in the 10 years 1942–52. More recent estimates give 1.5 per 1000.

This marked discrepancy in incidence is explained by our certain knowledge that the majority of hips which at birth show signs of instability will right themselves spontaneously. This spontaneous cure rate might be as high as 80 per cent (Solomon, 1973; Finlay, Maudesley and Busfield, 1967). Mackenzie (1972) wrote of his experiences running a special clinic for neonatal hip problems in the Aberdeen area. From a population of 76 675 live births 1671 infants were

71

referred to him. These referrals were because the hip was dislocated, dislocatable or stiff, i.e. showed significant limitation of abduction. Thus we had brought to our notice another state of the neonate's hip. Of each 100 abnormal hips referred to his clinic at birth, 78 were unstable and 22 stiff. If he did nothing and examined the same 100 infants again at 3 weeks old he found that 49 were normal, 27 were unstable and 24 were stiff. But these 24 stiff hips at 3 weeks old did not include all of the 22 that were stiff at birth; 11 came from that group but 13 came from the group that were unstable at birth!

The situation is confused by Williamson's report from Northern Ireland, 1972 stating that in the years 1962–63 no unstable hips were seen among 7959 live births, but in the years 1968–69 among 6838 live births there were 28 unstable hips requiring splintage. Mackenzie's chart says that if the femoral head moves on performing Barlow's test there is dislocation which requires splintage. On the other hand Barlow (1962) splints only dislocated hips and not those which he calls unstable or dislocatable because they show spontaneous recovery. These problems are further confused by consideration of the hip which gives a positive 'clunk' sign at birth but not at 5 to 7 days old. Mitchell (1972) believes that these should be splinted if the radiograph shows displacement, implying that without this evidence it is safe to leave the hip alone. Sharrard (1972) believes that these hips should be splinted for 8 weeks, and yet Barlow found a spontaneous recovery rate in abnormal hips of 58 per cent in the first $3\frac{1}{2}$ days. The purpose of splinting all abnormal hips in neonates is to treat effectively those which will not recover spontaneously. Barlow thinks this is 12 per cent of the hips which are unstable at birth.

Stanisavljevic (1964) wrote a monograph describing his findings and deductions from examining 6000 newborn babies and dissecting 300 hips of stillborn babies. His findings can only alarm those who thought they understood the problems if not the answers. He found 39 hips in 6000 babies which gave a positive Ortolani's sign. He believes this sign indicates a congenital hip subluxation and should be treated by a Frejka pillow for 3 months. Spontaneous improvement without treatment did not occur. Furthermore he found 5 dislocated hips among the 300 hips of stillborn infants that he dissected (why so many?). These did not show positive Ortolani's signs and neither had they limitation of abduction. Widespread confusion is no excuse for avoiding the issues.

The author's policy

Splinting all hips which appear unstable at birth is offering unnecessary treatment to 4 out of 5 infants. This would not matter if splintage was harmless, but it is not.

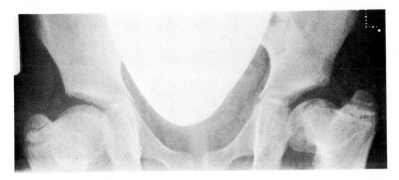

Figure 4.1. Bilateral coxa vara due to splinting an unstable left hip at birth

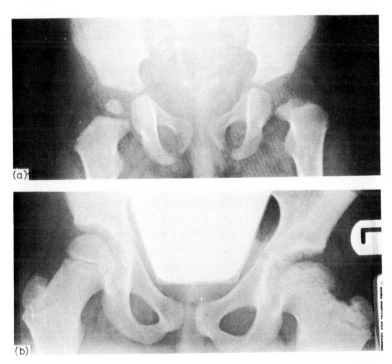

Figure 4.2. (a) Radiograph showing damage to the left femoral neck following treatment of left CDH. (b) The same hips at age 5 years

Figure 4.1 is the radiograph of a girl aged 7 years who at age 2 days was found to have a positive 'clunk' sign on the left. She was treated on a divaricator splint for 3 months. She now has coxa vara. *Figure 4.2* shows the hips at age 1 year and at age 5 years of another girl whose positive 'clunk' sign was splinted from age 2 days to age 3 months. There has been suppression of growth.

My policy is now to examine the newborn when the obstetrician or paediatrician has found suspicious hip signs. If I confirm a positive Ortolani sign I do nothing unless the same sign is found on the second examination at age 7 days. Then the hip is splinted.

The sign is positive if on abduction of the hip with pressure inwards at the greater trochanter there is a 'clunk' *in which the fatty tissue shakes.* Nothing else is unequivocal evidence that the femoral head was out of joint. This is so convincing a sign that if there is doubt among experienced examiners the sign is usually not positive. Hips giving this sign at age 1 day and *again at age 7 days* should be splinted. A hip which is reduced as the infant lies but can be coaxed out by pressure of the examiner's thumb backwards on the upper femur is a lax hip and I believe should be left alone. Such babies often lie at sleep with their hip in the classic frog position, a position never seen when the hip is dislocated.

Mackenzie (1972) does not treat any infants until the age of 3 weeks, believing that half will have improved spontaneously by then. Splintage at age 3 weeks is more difficult and more inconvenient for child and mother and has few advantages.

Infants escaping diagnosis

Mitchell (1972) found 4 dislocations presenting later among 31 961 infants born and examined in Edinburgh. Mackenzie (1972) found 30 missed dislocations from 28 426 infants born and examined in Aberdeen. In Glasgow about 15 per year are diagnosed later than the neonatal period and yet Ortolani's test is widely used. We must assume, in our present state of ignorance, that these dislocations have been missed at birth.

Stiff hips

Some dislocated hips are irreducible by the Ortolani method, but their number is small and their musculature tight. There remains a group of neonates in which one hip shows marked limitation of abduction (why always only one?) They do not give a positive 'clunk' test because it is not possible without causing pain to stretch the adductors sufficiently to perform the test fully. Finlay, Maudesley and Busfield include these in their 'normal' group. Mackenzie (1972) calls them 'stiff hips' and splints them like the unstable ones persisting at 3 weeks of age. We do not know the natural history of these stiff hips. I cannot splint these hips effectively so in mild ones I offer no treatment and where there is marked loss of abduction with apparent shortening I perform adductor tenotomy and immobilize

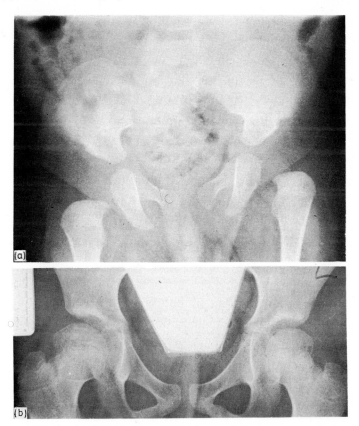

Figure 4.3. (a) Radiograph of the hips of a girl aged 2 weeks with limited adduction on the left. (b) The same hips 7 years later

the hips in an A-shaped plaster (groins to ankles) for 3 months. It is in this decision that radiographs help. *Figure 4.3a* is a strict antero-posterior view (patellae anterior, big toes tied together) of a girl aged 2 weeks who had tight adductors on both sides, left worse than right. (I find 'routine' radiographs of the hips of neonates impossible to interpret. It is essential to know the exact positions of the leg when the film is exposed. Radiographs taken with the leg in neutral rotation have meaning). The left leg has half-inch apparent shortening and excessive skin creases. Neither hip gave a positive 'clunk sign'. At 45 degrees the adductors prevented further abduction. We do not know what the future would hold for an infant so afflicted. The radiograph which because of the controlled position is interpretable shows marked adduction of the left hip and deficient acetabular roof development; thus dislocation is highly likely. I treated her by tenotomy and plaster in abduction for 6 months. *Figure 4.3b* shows the hips 7 years later.

In spite of the policies described, the Glasgow area—annual birth rate about 26 000—still presents us with 15 new cases of CDH per year which present after walking has begun. Finlay, Maudesley and Busfield (1967) were the first to point out that the neonate with a dislocated or dislocatable hip tended to be female, to present by the breech and to have a left-sided abnormality—facts which exactly parallel classic CDH. One is left with the conclusion that those who present later have either slipped through the neonatal diagnostic net or had dislocations at birth which were then irreducible.

Perhaps we studied neonatal CDH on a too superficial level. In 1962 we recognized the normal hip, the pre-natal dislocation and the hip giving a persistently positive 'clunk' sign. We now have to add two other types: the hip with a positive 'clunk' sign at birth becoming negative in the first week and the hip in joint but with marked loss of abduction. All five neonatal conditions require a different management and even when all five are recognized classic CDH will still present after walking begins. This event will be viewed by those still interested in the problems of established CDH without unrelieved sadness.

THE TREATMENT OF CONGENITAL DISLOCATION OF THE HIP IN THE AGE GROUP 1–4 YEARS

My reasons for dealing at length with this subject are threefold.

(1) Current textbooks describe the many differing ways of managing CDH but give little guidance on which to choose. It is difficult to find in the bewildering literature an account of the results produced by an exactly described course of treatment. Most long-term follow-up studies concern children treated in different ways or assessed without sufficient emphasis on the radiograph.

(2) Pelvic osteotomies have been used widely in recent years because of dissatisfaction with previous methods. Salter's marriage to innominate osteotomy admits of no impediments. His adoption of this operation is based on disappointment with previous treatments which did not include rotation osteotomy. It remains to

be seen whether rotation osteotomy in the course of treatment obviates the need for these more difficult operations.

(3) My experience is of 191 hips followed up from 8 to 18 years. During the years 1956–61 most of the controversial issues were faced and a course of treatment finally evolved that was used without change in 104 hips treated up to the end of 1966.

Attention is confined to typical dislocations in this age group. Hopefully dislocations presenting at over 4 years will remain rare.

Critique of previous papers

No attempt is made to review the whole literature. Certain significant papers are discussed which describe long-term results of significant numbers.

Müller and Seddon (1953) published a review of patients treated in the half century ending in 1940 at the Royal National Orthopaedic Hospital, London. Their paper is detailed and deserves close study. Although 889 cases were available the number actually analysed was 264, but only 130 whose treatment began between the ages 1 and 3 years were traced and examined at long-term follow-up. This review found reason for sober satisfaction with the results of closed reduction and 80 per cent of unilateral dislocations treated before age 3 years gave good results. These authors used, however, a grading scheme where it was possible for a hip result to be 'excellent' if it gave no pain and had a full range of movement but had a radiograph showing marked subluxation and gross deformity. The follow-up is in some cases less than 15 years so we cannot learn from this paper the end result. We are not told the details of the conservative management after reduction, rotation osteotomy was only done on 9 hips and in 5 of these was ineffective.

Wilkinson and Carter (1960) studied the results in 141 children where treatment, by others, began in the first 3 years of life. The reduction was either by manipulation under anaesthesia or by fixed skin traction in abduction. This was followed by 9–12 months' fixation in abduction and neutral rotation by either plaster or a harness. Their follow-up was from 4 to 10 years and their grades of result decided by radiographs. Grades 1 and 2 of the 5 used were considered to be hips unlikely to develop arthritis. A close correlation was found in unilateral cases between the result of this conservative treatment and the slope of the opposite acetabular roof such that girls with normal opposite acetabula gave 40 successful results out of 54. They suggest that early operative treatment is indicated for unilateral cases where the opposite acetabular is shallow. They do not describe the results of such a policy. Rotation osteotomy was not used in their series and they state, 'If anteversion exists it cannot by itself be more than an exceptional cause of failure of conservative treatment.' Twenty-four out of 94 girls with unilateral dislocations had their opposite acetabular angle more than 2 standard deviations above the mean. Conservative treatment of the dislocated hip in these 24 gave 16 failures, 5 intermediate results and 3 successes. We cannot assess fully this contribution unless we are told why 8 did not fail or whether the opposite acetabular slope remained the same throughout childhood.

Mackenzie, Seddon and Trevor (1960) report 88 per cent satisfactory results in unilateral cases under age 3 years treated by frame reduction followed by 10 months in Batchelor plaster in full internal rotation and then freedom. They then performed 'preventive acetabuloplasty' on hips which were clinically normal but were thought likely to subluxate; 30.5 per cent were so treated. Another 7.1 per cent received corrective acetabuloplasty. Both operations are reported to give good results such that they recommend no haste in operating on a defective acetabulum. They assume, as do most authors from Wiberg (1939) onwards, that a radiological appearance of acetabular dysplasia foretells disaster and must therefore be treated surgically. It does not seem rational to hold the child's hip in full internal rotation for 10 months and then allow free movement. As rotation osteotomy was only performed on 24.8 per cent of their hips over 75 per cent will have the anteversion, considered so important for the first 10 months of post-reduction development, uncorrected. Their results are similar to those of Wilkinson and Carter (1960) from the same city, where abduction and neutral rotation were used. If we knew how this is possible we should understand more about the child's hip joint.

These papers concentrated on the reduction of the dislocation and its effect on the late result rather than on the whole treatment. Smith et al. (1968) do the same. Their paper describes results assessed at an average of age 31 years of 75 dislocations in 53 children reduced at between 1 and 8 months. Measuring the radiograph when immobilization was discontinued disclosed that 21 of the 75 had theoretically perfect reductions but only 7 of these were normal at follow-up.

Somerville (1953) stated that, 'The results of conservative treatment show that in about one-third the results are reasonably good, while in about two-thirds they are unreasonably bad.' In consequence he devised a safer, smaller open reduction than hitherto. Then he and Scott (Somerville and Scott, 1957) advocated a direct approach to CDH. This consists of frame reduction, arthrography, excision of the limbus and rotation osteotomy on all hips. This last operation had had a bad press up to this time. Their course of treatment lasted 14 weeks and their results' assessment was based solely on the radiographs, as they realized that to introduce pain and range of movement into a 10-year result was misleading. 'Excellent' and 'Good' final results were considered unlikely to give further trouble.

Salter (1961) looked again at the problem. He searched for a cause of instability after reduction in a dislocation at over 18 months and found it in the inclination of the whole acetabulum. He states, 'By about 18 months normal osseous development of the acetabulum and femoral head is no longer assured even by prolonged retention of the reduced hip in a stable position' and 'Rotation osteotomy does not always prevent upwards and lateral subluxation'. But of the 13 earlier result studies he quotes none has used rotation osteotomy extensively. The operation he advises is one which reduces the acetabulum over the femoral head. Innominate osteotomy is performed at the same time as open reduction of the hip. This three-plane correction is now widely used. Since 1968 the British and American literature on CDH in this age group has included many reports on this operation and other pelvic osteotomies (Pemberton, 1961; Chiari, 1955) as if the standard treatments of this disorder, upon which most of us were brought up, have been proved inadequate.

The choices available

Having familiarized himself with the literature the clinician must decide five basic questions.

(1) The method of reduction and whether to use arthrography.

(2) The type of open reduction to use and its indication.

(3) The place of acetabular reconstruction and its timing.

(4) The importance of anteversion and its correction by femoral osteotomy.

(5) Whether or not to abandon classic methods and perform open reduction and innominate osteotomy on all true CDH in this age group.

Evolution of present policy

An account of my reasoning on the above issues may help others facing these problems. I described open reduction early in the discourse because important conclusions were drawn from the findings, but it is only used in one-third of reductions.

The 'direct approach' of Somerville and Scott (1957) was attractive and convincing and was used in the early years of clinical responsibility. Dissatisfaction with some of the steps in their 14-week programme plus evidence from open reductions caused changes to be made. Frame reduction proved time-consuming and inaccurate. Three to 4 weeks were spent in getting the femoral head opposite to the acetabulum in a child who at the time of diagnosis was older than desirable. It was often necessary to perform a final manipulation under anaesthesia to get the head reduced. Frame reduction would be indicated if the incidence of osteochondritis were significantly lessened or if this complication marred the end result. I found no such evidence.

Salter and Kostuik (1969) showed that the hip position producing least strain on the vascular structures in a reduced dislocation is one of flexion and moderate abduction. It did not seem rational to attempt reduction by traction in extension particularly as evidence suggests that the hip dislocates by extension in the newborn.

Arthrography was used in 54 hips, mostly in children over age 2 years where it was important to distinguish between subluxation and dislocation. When arthrographic changes suggested an inturned limbus, 'a globular rag turned into the acetabulum' (Somerville and Scott, 1957), an open reduction was performed. At operation I did not see a fibrocartilaginous structure occluding the acetabulum enabling dye to lie on both sides as was suggested by the radiographs. The 'limbus' was plastered to the superoposterior segment of the socket. It could not be left behind and it was not the only bar to reduction as Somerville had suggested. I was also concerned with the duration of treatment. Two hips treated along the Somerville–Scott lines both re-dislocated about 6 months after the end of the 14 weeks' treatment.

In consequence modifications began to creep in. By 1960 I had experience of 38 fully annotated open reductions performed mostly on children in their third year of life. If the anatomical changes in younger children are similar to those seen at open operation, and we presume that they are, then deductions can be made as to what steps are necessary to place the femoral head deeply into the floor of the acetabulum—the most important part of any treatment programme. My present policy is based on theoretical considerations plus important evidence from open reduction, the lessons from which influence the method of closed reduction for younger children whose anatomical changes are not so marked.

Description of open reduction
A routine Smith–Petersen approach is used dividing the origin of rectus femoris and developing the interval between the psoas tendon and the inferior capsule. The capsule is opened after cleaning its superior, anterior and inferior surfaces by a cut parallel and close to its iliac attachment not transversely as described in Campbell's

Operative Orthopaedics (1971). The femoral head is smooth, healthy and of such a size that it will go into a normal acetabulum. It may not be spherical. The femoral neck is always anteverted such that to reduce it requires between 70 degrees and 100 degrees of internal rotation. The ligamentum teres is now cut from the head and followed down through a glistening, pouting orifice which resembles the cervix uteri as seen through a speculum. This orifice is bounded superoposteriorly by the thickened fibrocartilaginous limbus and antero-inferiorly by capsule reflected over a thickened psoas tendon and transverse ligament. Traction on and removal of the proximal end of the ligamentum teres enables a blunt hook to be inserted beneath the lower edge of the limbus. This hook is moved forcibly forwards. The leg is now flexed to 90 degrees and externally rotated so that the hook can be moved backwards to free the edge of the limbus. Taking the handle of the hook inferiorly makes its blunt point penetrate the outer acetabular edge between limbus and articular cartilage. This plane of cleavage is opened and the fibrocartilaginous limbus is removed. The inferior capsule is pulled inferiorly. If there is resistance it is cut and the tendon of psoas which causes resistance is resected. The inferior capsule is pulled inferiorly at least 1 inch. Remnants of fat, limbus and ligament are now scraped out of the true acetabulum with a 1-inch gauge covered by a swab using a rotatory motion. These steps reveal an acetabulum which is surprisingly normal both in shape and in cartilaginous covering. Traction is now put on the leg and in abduction and full internal rotation the head reduces so that its articular cartilage completely disappears from view. If there is any springiness tending to eject the femoral head the inferior dissection and excision is incomplete. The cut in the capsule closes itself in this position and the wound is closed after re-attachment of rectus femoris. A plaster spica is now applied in abduction and full internal rotation.

These findings have been invariable in 51 operations.

Inferences

(1) Reduction of congenital dislocation by non-operative means must relax the tissues which have caused the head to lie superiorly. Thus the position of extension and abduction as used on a frame is unsuitable for this problem. The leg must be flexed above a right angle, the trochanter lifted forwards and guided inwards as the thigh is abducted. This guided manipulation has fallen into disrepute but is logical if the course of the ligamentum teres is visualized.

(2) It was impossible to get the femoral head seated deeply in older children without surgical division or strong retraction of the structures occluding the inferior half of the acetabulum. Thus if open

operation were necessary the limited 'limbectomy' approach of Somerville and Scott (1957) was not adequate in my hands.

(3) I found a lack of agreement between pre-operative arthrograms and the findings at operation. As I do not know the exact structures giving the shadows on arthrography I think its value in determining which hips should be opened is exaggerated.

(4) Marked femoral anteversion was invariable; thus a long period in full internal rotation is necessary for the femoral head to exert its deepening effect on the acetabulum, then rotation osteotomy must follow.

Manipulative reduction

I now attempt reduction under anaesthesia as soon as a diagnosis is made. The technique described is an Ortolani sign under anaesthesia and will reduce a dislocation; with the manipulator having a mental picture of the head going along its correct path, the greater trochanter will sink inwards with a thud, similar to a classic Ortolani sign. On abduction in full flexion the adductors will become tight. When they are standing out subcutaneously the abduction should be lessened. At about 40 degrees abduction the hip will dislocate posteriorly just like the infant with CDH. It is again reduced, tenotomy of the adductors is performed and a full Lorenz first position plaster is applied with the knees each about 10 degrees anterior to the coronal plane of the body and the body and the hips flexed above a right angle. After this manipulation a radiograph is taken in the position of supposed reduction.

In typical CDH at age 1–4 years the decision whether or not to perform open reduction is made upon the sensation of reduction and the appearance of the post-reduction radiograph. This should show concentric reduction i.e. the acetabulum and the outline of the femoral capital epiphysis should be parallel. The femoral neck should point at the inferior quadrant of the acetabulum and the head should not be standing away. If there is real doubt about the reduction as revealed by the sensation of touch and hearing or about the radiograph then open reduction should be carried out as described. The hip can then be placed in internal rotation and abduction because of the excisions performed.

Management after reduction

Three months in a Lorenz frog plaster seems a compromise between the too rapid adoption of the internal rotation position with loss of congruity and possible pelvitrochanteric adhesion formation that can delay mobilization of the hip that spends too long in the frog position.

After 3 months the legs are gently rolled into neutral rotation (under anaesthesia) maintaining abduction as before and plaster is again applied over legs and lower abdomen. After a further 1 month this plaster is removed and internal rotation is achieved by rolling inwards the affected leg, the knees are flexed and a Batchelor plaster applied. An estimate of the degree of anteversion present can be made from the post-reduction radiograph in the frog position. As this picture shows a lateral view of the femoral shaft any angle that the neck makes with the shaft is the angle of anteversion. Its exact measurement is not important. It is almost always significant and the hip should be placed in as much internal rotation as can be gained without force. In a small proportion of cases internal rotation is not necessary. If there is doubt then at this stage, 4 months after reduction, an anteroposterior radiograph is taken in neutral rotation and again with the leg in full internal rotation. If on the second film the femoral neck appears significantly longer then this position is used. The Batchelor plaster remains on for 3 months. Movements of the hip aid acetabular development and dispersion of soft tissue. At 7 months after reduction subtrochanteric derotation osteotomy is performed.

Technique of osteotomy

This method, learned from Somerville 1957–58, is better than that of Crego or Platou as described in Campbell (1971).

A lateral exposure with the leg in full internal rotation is used. When the upper 3 inches of the femoral shaft have been exposed, a No. 8, four-hole plate is applied to the outer surface. A guide-wire is placed horizontally through the second hole from the top to penetrate the lateral cortex and engage the medial cortex. A second guide-wire is now inserted vertically at 90 degrees to the first. It pierces the anterior cortex at a point in line with the third plate hole and engages the posterior cortex. These guide-wires are now at 90 degrees to each other and separated by the exact distance between screw holes two and three of the plate. The plate is then threaded off the upper guide-wire and the bone divided with a handsaw between the guide-wires. After complete transverse division of the bone the upper fragment is kept in full internal rotation by control from the guide-wire and the lower fragment is then externally rotated until the guide-wires are parallel and horizontal. The plate is then threaded over both wires which now occupy holes two and three of the plate. Screws are now applied in holes one and four, the guide-wires are removed and screws inserted into holes two and three. This gives approximately 90 degrees derotation. In some children the lower leg is now in slight external rotation. The wound is closed and a single hip spica applied on the affected leg, holding it in abduction and in the degree of rotation that the plating has determined. After 6 weeks this plaster is removed and a final A-shaped plaster, groin to ankle, is applied to both legs for a final 6 weeks, making 10 months from first reduction. At this time the outpatient attendance consists of removing all plaster and instructing the parents to allow the child to do exactly as she likes. Some will stand immediately, some will shuffle for several weeks before standing. No physiotherapy or other encouragement is used.

If reduction is by open operation an internal rotation hip spica is used and 6 weeks after operation the sutures are removed and a Batchelor plaster is applied again in full internal rotation and retained as for manipulated hips for 3 more months.

This treatment is now used on all hips of children aged between 1 and 4 years which satisfy Somerville's definition of 'typical dislocations', i.e. are not demonstrably associated with any other pathological state.

The results it can be expected to produce and the reasons why it was adopted must now be considered.

Results and grading

The experience here reported is a personal series of 170 children with congenital dislocation of the hip treated between 1 and 4 years of age. Fourteen children have been excluded because in spite of personal retention of the records and radiographs and diligent attention to follow-up, they have been lost or their final radiograph has been unobtainable. This leaves 156 children who had 191 dislocated hips.

They have been divided into two groups.

Group I

This group was treated between 1956 and 1960 and comprises 87 hips in 71 children. The children have now reached skeletal maturity (minimum follow-up 14 years). They were treated during the evolution of the present programme. The results are 68 (78.1 per cent) 'good' and 19 'bad' hips.

Group II

This group was treated between 1961 and 1966 in exactly the way described in this chapter and comprises 104 hips in 85 children. The results are 93 good (89.4 per cent) and 11 bad hips.

All children are mobile and active; none have significant pain. The grading concentrates solely on the radiographs and is simplified to make two categories—good and bad.

The follow-up radiographs are studied. Some are normal hips, others show blemishes or severe incongruities. A result is graded good if the femoral head is two-thirds or more covered by the acetabulum. Shenton's line must either be normal or show no worsening on annual radiographs. The acetabular roof must show improvement of its coverage of the femoral head on annual radiographs and its outer lip must be horizontal. The joint must be congruous.

This definition comprises Somerville's good and excellent groups and Grades 1 and 2 of the Wilkinson–Carter paper. It agrees with Severin's (1941) classification of radiological results and corresponds closely to the classification excellent and good used by Salter (1974).

A bad result, on the other hand, will show a progressive break in Shenton's line, inadequate development of the acetabular roof or a worsening picture on annual radiographs.

Up to half an inch shortening due to coxa vara is acceptable in the good grade provided the femoral head and acetabulum are parallel, i.e. their outlines are segments of circles with the same centre. Shortening from subluxation, of course, or coxa vara with a flattened

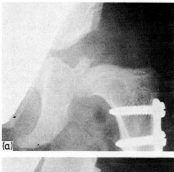
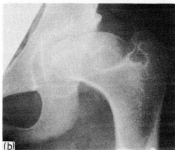

Figure 4.4. An 11-year result of left CDH marred by osteochondritis

head renders the result bad (*Figure 4.4*). My best results are in Group II: 89.4 per cent excellent or good from 104 hips. This is slightly inferior to Salter and Dubos' recent figures (1974) where 93.6 per cent are excellent or good from 110 similar hips. It is reasonable to expect these percentages in both series to give no further hip trouble.

Deviations from accepted teaching

Frame reduction

Seventeen children in Group I whose dislocations were reduced on the Wingfield–Morris frame were compared with the next 17 similar cases whose hips were manipulated. There were 5 cases of oesteochondritis, 2 after frame reduction and 3 following manipulation. In none of these was the end result marred by this complication. In the whole series of 191 hips osteochondritis was seen in 23 hips. In 2 only was there permanent deformity of the femoral head sufficient to categorize the end result as bad (*Figure 4.4*).

In both cases the capital epiphysis was split into two parts whereas in the 21 hips where the osteochondritis improved the fragmentation was generalized throughout the epiphysis (*see Figure 4.19*).

Frame reduction did not seem, to me, justifiable.

Arthrography

There were 4 technical failures but no complications among the 54 hips injected. In order to find out whether my lack of confidence in interpreting the radiographs was or was not well founded I ran 2 test cases in which I ignored findings which would earlier have led me to perform open reduction.

> *Figure 4.5a* is an arthrogram of the left hip of a girl aged 1 year 7 months. No significance was attached to the appearance shown. Closed reduction and frog plaster were used for 3 months followed by 1 month in neutral rotation and then 3 months in Batchelor plaster in internal rotation. *Figure 4.5b* shows the position at this stage just before a 90 degree derotation osteotomy. *Figure 4.5c* shows the same hip 11 years later.

The other case was similar. This evidence plus the knowledge that complications from injecting iodine-containing solutions into the hip are not unknown suggested that the value of arthrography in deciding which hips should be opened was exaggerated. Its use for this purpose was abandoned.

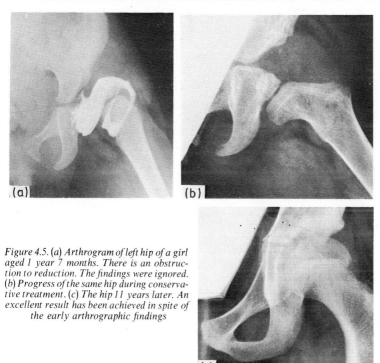

Figure 4.5. (a) Arthrogram of left hip of a girl aged 1 year 7 months. There is an obstruction to reduction. The findings were ignored. (b) Progress of the same hip during conservative treatment. (c) The hip 11 years later. An excellent result has been achieved in spite of the early arthrographic findings

Open reduction

Reduction of the 87 hips in Group I was achieved by closed methods in 49 and open methods in 38. Of these 38, 11 were treated by the arthrotomy approach of Somerville and Scott (1957). Two of these 11 caused concern. *Figure 4.6a* shows the position achieved in a typical CDH after frame reduction, arthrography, excision of the limbus and, 2 months later, rotation osteotomy. All looked satisfactory. Mobilization was allowed 14 weeks after reduction. Four years later there was evidence of superior subluxation and deficient acetabular roof formation (*Figure 4.6b*).

This event constitutes the fascination of CDH. Many hips which turn out normal appear identical to *Figure 4.6a* at the same stage. Did this case and another similar one fail because the arthrotomy and excision of the limbus was insufficient for complete reduction or because the 14 weeks' treatment advised by Somerville was too short? Both factors were changed and full open reduction, as described, was performed on hips which gave an unsatisfactory manipulative reduction or a post-reduction radiograph which showed any

88

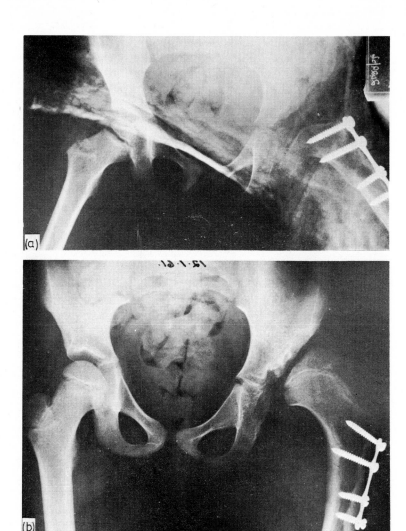

Figure 4.6. (a) Open reduction by Somerville technique followed by rotation osteotomy. The position looks satisfactory. (b) The same hips 4 years later. There has been recurrence of dislocation on the left side

degree of 'standing away'. Further experience led me to understand less about pre-reduction arthrographic shadows and more about the importance of exposing the whole acetabulum and paying attention to the inferior part and the obstructions therein. As pre-reduction arthrography was done less often the incidence of open reduction declined and in the second series, Group II of 104 hips, reduction was achieved by manipulation in 80 and by open reduction in 24. Thus in the entire series of 191 hips there were 62 open reductions, 11 by the Somerville technique and 51 by the bigger operation.

Rotation osteotomy

To decide how many hips in the age group 1–4 years at reduction required rotation osteotomy it was necessary again to run a test case. Other writers less emphatic about anteversion than Somerville and Scott (1957) had suggested that this deformity might be due to the Batchelor plaster used. Others had had satisfactory results correcting anteversion rarely or not at all. Accordingly a typical case, well reduced, was followed through the usual course of treatment but given only 6 weeks in the internal rotation (IR) position and then 4 months in abduction and neutral rotation.

Figure 4.7a shows the left hip of a girl aged 18 months, before treatment. The position after the period in IR is shown in *Figure 4.7b* and *Figure 4.7c* shows the appearance in abduction and neutral rotation. No osteotomy was performed. This was a mistake. The position 11 years after reduction is shown in *Figure 4.7d;* the result is bad.

I have not seen a position like *Figure 4.7b* give other than an excellent result when rotation osteotomy has been performed and I conclude therefore that the poor result is due solely to its absence.

This operation was performed on 189 of the 191 hips in this series. Study of the early cases showed that acetabular roof growth was accelerated by the osteotomy. Hips which other authors would treat by acetabular surgery seemed to respond to osteotomy alone.

Pelvic operations

No innominate osteotomies and only one acetabuloplasty, which did not work, were performed on these patients. It was important to see whether rotation osteotomy alone would produce stability without embarking on more difficult operations. No previous paper had discussed this question.

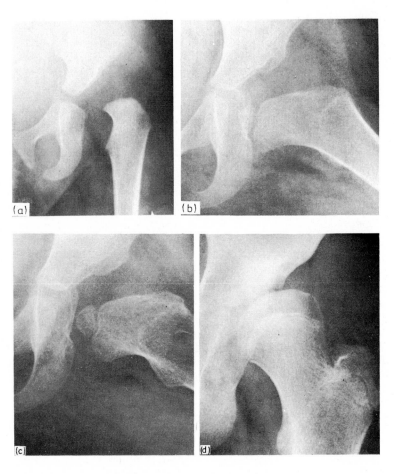

Figure 4.7. (a) Left CDH in a girl aged 18 months. The position in internal rotation (b) did not differ much from the position in neutral rotation (c). Rotation osteotomy was not performed. (d) shows the bad result 11 years later

Results

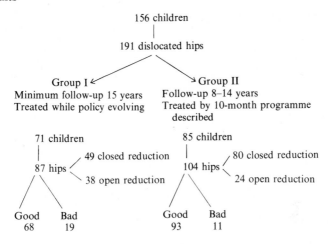

156 children

191 dislocated hips

Group I — Group II

Minimum follow-up 15 years — Follow-up 8–14 years
Treated while policy evolving — Treated by 10-month programme described

71 children — 85 children

87 hips — 49 closed reduction / 38 open reduction — 104 hips — 80 closed reduction / 24 open reduction

Good 68 — Bad 19 — Good 93 — Bad 11

Final results (assessed from radiographs at follow-up)   Good 161
Bad   30

Results judged from radiographs at end of 10 months' treatment (the post-treatment radiograph)

Encouraging—Acet. roof development beginning	125
Discouraging—Subluxation or other bad feature evident	17
Problem hips—No acet. roof development and yet no subluxation	49

Ultimate fate of the 49 problem hips at follow-up   Good 36
Bad 13

    Of the 161 hips which at follow-up were graded good 125 had begun to show at least a trace of acetabular roof development during the course of the 10 months' treatment such that on the anteroposterior (AP) radiograph taken when the last plaster was removed— the post-treatment (PT) radiograph—there was not much doubt that the acetabulum was responding. In 49, however, no such beginning had occurred. These 49, the problem hips, were left alone.

Effect of sex of child on end result

Patients	Number of typical CDH	Result at follow-up 8–18 years	
		Good	Bad
23 boys	26	22	4
133 girls	165	139	26
159	191	161	30

Effect of age at reduction on end result

This study concerns children with typical CDH reduced at between 12 and 48 months of age. In Group II, all of whom had the same treatment, the average age of the 10 children who gave 11 bad results was 20.8 months. The average age of the whole group was 17.3 months at reduction.

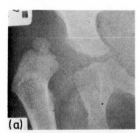

(a)

Figure 4.8 A good result of the management described in the text. (a) Right CDH at age 16 months. (b) The position just before the end of 10 months' treatment. (c) The hip at age 14 years

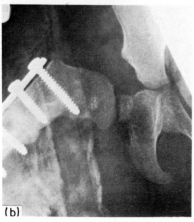

(b)

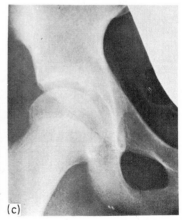

(c)

The failures of treatment

Eighty-seven dislocations in 71 children in Group I all have a minimum follow-up of 15 years. Although their treatment was not identical their skeletal maturity at follow-up makes them separate from Group II.

Study of the bad results in Group I

On the criteria described 68 are good and 19 are bad. A typical good result is shown in *Figure 4.8*. This girl's hip, reduced at 1 year 4 months, was treated exactly as outlined earlier under conservative treatment.

Osteochondritis occurred in 5 hips but healed spontaneously and did not cause any of the 19 failures.

Two children with 3 dislocated hips also had scoliosis, in 1 case congenital, the other idiopathic. All these 3 hips were bad results because the acetabulum did not mould to cover the reduced femoral head. Seven hips were failures because the open reduction had been inadequate. One failure occurred in a mentally retarded boy, the other 8 failures occurred in apparently normal children whose reduction was thought to be satisfactory but whose acetabular roof failed to grow over the femoral head.

Causes of 19 Bad Results in 87 Hips
Followed to Skeletal Maturity

Presence of other abnormalities	4
Technical failure of reduction or after-treatment	7
Inadequate acetabular growth after successful reduction	8
	19

Comment

None of the children having the 68 good results had any other abnormality except one with a cleft palate.

Some, if not all, of the 7 failures of reduction were due to operative inexperience.

Some of the failures of acetabular roof growth were thought to be due to too brief a period of treatment.

All the failures had declared themselves by 5 years after reduction; thus, using the criteria of good and bad described, assessment at 5–8 years after reduction is valuable.

In the light of these results and the experiences described with other techniques the routine of treatment became established which was used without alteration from 1961 onwards.

The Group II Series

This group all had the treatment described. There were 104 hips in 85 children which when assessed on follow-up in 1974 from 8 to 14 years after reduction gave 93 good and 11 bad results. For the reasons given it is expected that these categories will remain.

Causes of 11 Bad Results in 104 Hips

Presence of other abnormalities	2
Technical failure of open reduction	2
Osteochondritis leading to deformity	2
Inadequate acetabular growth after successful reduction	5
	11

Study of the bad results in Group II

In 2 children aged 2 and $2\frac{1}{2}$ years the tissues were too tight at open reduction for the springiness already mentioned to be overcome when the head was rotated into the socket. Although 1 was a boy, no pre-operative suggestion of this difficulty was found. They failed by the head assuming the bulging shape which Somerville had found was associated with poor results in 13 out of 33 hips with this deformity; the bulging head had moved laterally 3–6 months after reduction and then subluxated (*Figure 4.9*).

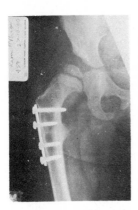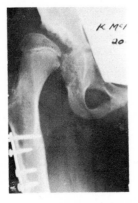

Figure 4.9. Subluxation of the left hip 4 years after treatment. The bulging head is shown

One failure occurred in a girl with a congenital lumbosacral defect and a paralytic foot on the other side. Another failure occurred in a girl with club foot. Two developed irrecoverable osteochondritis that rendered the joint surface not parallel. The largest group, however, were, like Group I, those whose reduction appeared satisfactory and yet failed because of inadequate growth of the acetabular roof.

Apart then from the presence of other abnormalities thought unimportant on first examination, the cause of failure in well-reduced congenital dislocations lies in the acetabular roof.

Acetabular growth—the vital factor—the enigma

This structure determines whether the hip will be normal or just good. Every writer on this subject has a group of results which are normal hips whose prognosis is known. When we introduce a 'good' group it is a second best, a hip which we assume will remain trouble-free if our definition of 'good' is rigidly applied but there must be doubt. Provided that we can get the femoral head deeply into the socket and hold it there for a lengthy period avoiding iatrogenic complications in both of these processes, we are entirely dependent upon acetabular roof growth for the end result. If the roof did not form in outwardly facing acetabula the treatment would be innominate osteotomy. If the roof showing poor ossification throughout the course of treatment always remained defective then the last step of treatment would be acetabuloplasty. There are powerful advocates of both policies. I know of no firm evidence to guide the clinician.

Studying the radiograph taken after 10 months' treatment, the PT radiograph, the result had declared itself good or bad in 142 out of 191. In 49 hips there was no acetabular response and yet no subluxation or redislocation. With no further treatment 36 of these 49 became good at follow-up and 13 worsened. Their prognosis could be surmised 1 year after treatment finished and was definite within 2 years.

Examples have been shown where superior progression of the femoral head has resulted from inadequate open reduction (*Figure 4.6b*), and from failure to correct anteversion (*Figure 4.7c*), but if these were the only causes of defective acetabular roof formation the late results in a future series should, by their elimination, be uniformly good, but the acetabular roof was inadequate at follow-up in 13 hips in this series where neither cause applied.

The problem hips

Forty-nine hips showed no acetabular roof growth whatever on the 10-month radiograph, the PT radiograph, and yet without any

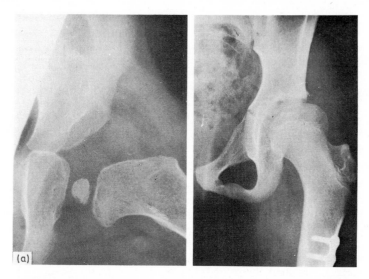

Figure 4.10. A problem hip that did well. (a) is the post-treatment radiograph showing no acetabular response after 10 months. (b) is the same hip 12 years later

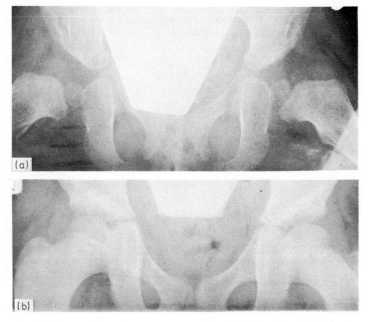

Figure 4.11. (a) Bilateral CDH in the 'problem hip' group. (b) Good result 12 years later

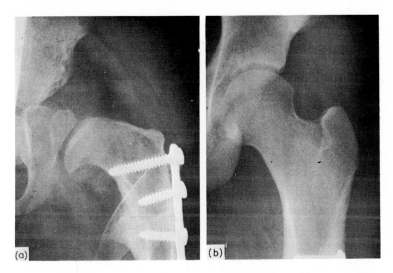

Figure 4.12. The PT radiograph shows no acetabular roof growth (a) and yet without treatment the hip is normal 15 years later (b)

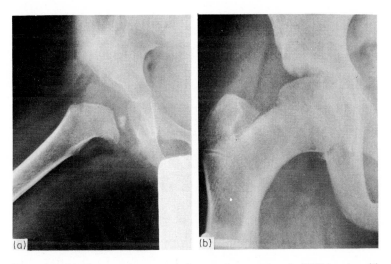

Figure 4.13. (a) The appearances just before rotation osteotomy in CDH in a boy. (b) The hip is normal 14 years later

treatment 36 improved to satisfy the criteria of good and 13 did not. The Figures (*a*) in the four paired radiographs (*Figures 4.10–4.13*) are all anteroposterior, PT radiographs. They are from this group of 49 problem hips which differ from the other 142 in that the prognosis is unknown. All the children were allowed to walk and no further treatment was given. The (*b*) figures are their follow-up radiographs 10–14 years later. All are 'good' hips. It is unlikely that any will give rise to further hip trouble. The PT radiographs, however, show features which many surgeons would consider altering by operation. Presumably Mackenzie, Seddon and Trevor (1960) would perform acetabuloplasty when seeing such changes. Wiberg and Howarth would turn down a shelf. Salter would not be in this position.

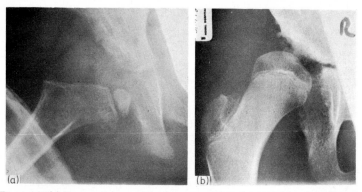

Figure 4.14.(a) No acetabular roof development on the radiograph taken 7 months after reduction. (b) 10 years later the hip is unsatisfactory in spite of rotation osteotomy

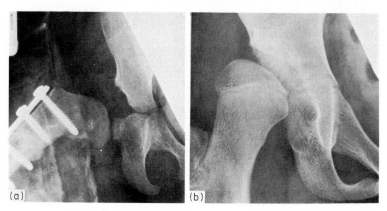

Figure 4.15. (a) The appearances after rotation osteotomy are satisfactory. (b) 12 years later there is subluxation

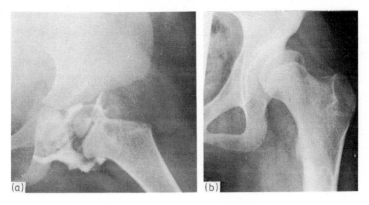

Figure 4.16. (a) The appearances after 7 months' treatment showing a satisfactory cartilagenous acetabulum. (b) 12 years later the result is bad

The above set of paired figures (*Figures 4.14–4.16*) show the PT radiograph (again the (*a*) figure) of another 3 hips from these 49. The (*b*) figure is again the follow-up radiograph. All 3 are bad results. If one offers acetabular surgery to all problem hips to avoid failure from this cause my results suggest that such surgery would be unecessary in about 70 per cent of hips (i.e. 36 out of 49). And yet I can see no factor present in the child or the radiograph which gives a guide to the future.

Inference

Acetabular roof growth is genetically determined.

Accurate deep reduction, then placing the femoral neck by rotation osteotomy such that its long axis is pointing to the floor of the acetabulum, is in some way a stimulus to growth of the acetabular roof such that 1 year after reduction 142 out of 191 will show a response but 49 (25 per cent) will not. If left alone about 70 per cent of these will improve and 30 per cent worsen.

We must now consider seven possibly relevant factors.

Inferior placement of the head

Two hips which showed a total absence of acetabular roof formation on the 10-month radiograph and did well appeared to have the femoral head lower in the acetabulum than usual. *Figure 4.17* shows the position just before rotation osteotomy and the same hip 11 years later.

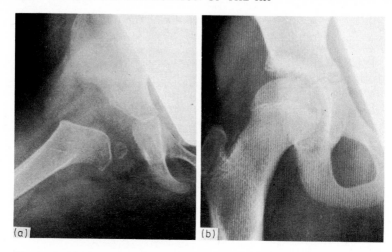

Figure 4.17. (a) The position just before rotation osteotomy. The femoral head was low
in the acetabulum. (b) A good 11-year result followed

Another problem hip from the group of 49 now under discussion
showed on the 10-month radiograph perhaps the worst acetabulum
of them all. This hip was treated by derotation osteotomy of 110
degrees (*Figure 4.18*). This pointed the femoral neck to the inferior
part of the socket. The acetabular roof ossified well. This feature is
not always associated with a good result. *Figures 4.14* and *4.15* show
hips with an equally low femoral head and identical treatment but
they had bad end results.

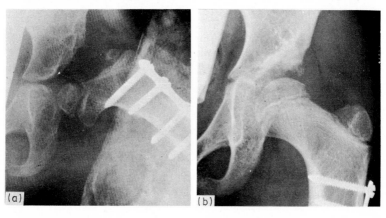

Figure 4.18. (a) A very poor acetabulum on the PT radiograph, but a low femoral head.
(b) Good result 13 years later

Sclerotic changes

As previously stated osteochondritis of the femoral head did not mar the end result in these patients except in 2 hips where the head became split into two fragments. *Figure 4.19a* shows the position in a Batchelor plaster 7 months after reduction in a girl aged 2 years. The whole head appears dense and the acetabular roof has shown no ossification. She received rotation osteotomy and 10 years later the hip was normal (*Figure 4.19b*). Sclerosis of the acetabular roof was said by Mackenzie, Seddon and Trevor (1960) to indicate acetabuloplasty to avoid a poor result. This feature has not necessarily

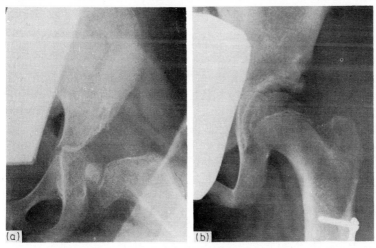

Figure 4.19. A 10-year result graded 'good' (b) although there was osteochondritis of the femoral head (a)

been associated with bad results. *Figure 4.20a* shows both hips in internal rotation of a girl with bilateral CDH 7 months after reduction by manipulation. Both roofs are sloping and show slight sclerotic change. She received bilateral rotation osteotomy and 7 years later the hips were good (*Figure 4.20b*).

Similarly a unilateral case (*Figure 4.21*) from among the 49 problem hips shows many features suggesting a poor outcome including sclerosis of the acetabular roof (*a*). Twelve years later the hip is normal (*b*).

The inclination of the upper femoral epiphyseal plate

Some hips have a straight epiphyseal line making the head hemispherical while others have a crescentic head as the epiphyseal line

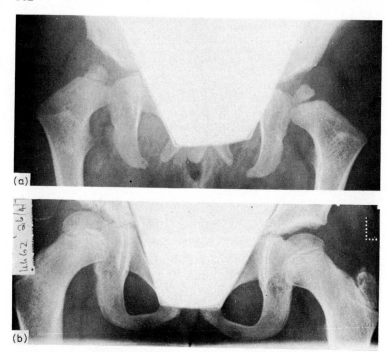

Figure 4.20. Both hips in internal rotation of a girl with a bilateral CDH 7 months after reduction (a). The 7-year result (b)

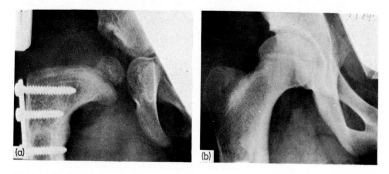

Figure 4.21. Total absence of acetabular roof growth on the 10-month radiograph (a) and yet 12 years later an excellent hip (b)

is the segment of a circle. Neither feature means anything in the end result of CDH.

Coxa valga and vara

Coxa valga is undesirable. It is a constant feature of the 3 failures shown (*Figures 4.14, 4.15,* and *4.16*). It is also seen in some of the good results (*Figure 4.20*).

A valgus neck can result from a hip looking varus at the end of treatment (*Figure 4.21*) or in one whose neck shaft angle is normal. *Figure 4.22* shows the position after treatment of a girl whose hip

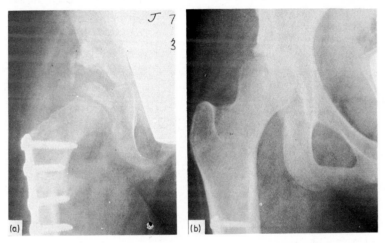

Figure 4.22. (a) The position after treatment of a girl aged 2 years treated by full open reduction and acetabuloplasty. (b) The 13-year result was graded 'bad'

was reduced by open reduction and prophylactic acetabuloplasty, the only one in the series. The outlook seemed good and yet 13 years later the roof was worse than on many not so treated.

Coxa vara on the other hand seems desirable. In cases where the end result has shown coxa vara sufficient to justify subtrochanteric abduction osteotomy (4 in this series) the PT radiograph has shown the capital epiphysis to be in two parts (*Figure 4.4*). Coxa vara with an intact femoral head has always resulted in a good hip at follow-up.

Femoral head standing away

The decision whether to reduce the hip by open operation is now made by the sensation of manipulative reduction and the radiograph taken thereafter. It is impossible to be dogmatic about this radiograph. As one's experience of open reduction grows one is happier to perform it if the post-reduction radiograph is anything short of perfect. This series, however, has produced surprises. *Figure 4.23a* shows a hip 6 months after full open reduction in which I had seen the cartilaginous head disappear deeply into the cleaned socket. The radiograph suggests soft-tissue obstruction which I know is not there—the result was good. It is when one sees radiographs like this after manipulative reduction that one is tempted to operate. *Figure 4.17* shows the position 4 months after a convincing manipulative reduction in which the head had been placed deeply in the socket. The anteroposterior view is of the hip in internal rotation just before application of the Batchelor plaster. Rotation osteotomy

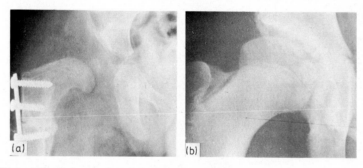

Figure 4.23. A surprising 'good' result 12 years after open reduction in a boy aged 2 years (b). The radiograph 6 months after reduction (a) looks appalling

followed this and 14 years later the hip was normal. But a girl whose radiograph (*Figure 4.14*), showed better seating of the femoral head at the same stage went on to fail, for no explicable reason.

Thus both arthrography and post-reduction radiographs can be misleading.

The shape of the opposite acetabulum

I have described 30 bad results in 191 hips, 19 in Group I and 11 in Group II. Twenty of these 30 failures were in unilateral dislocations. Seven of these 20 failures in unilateral cases were due to deficient acetabular roof formation and in 6 of the bilateral cases this was the only cause found. If we look at the shape of the opposite acetabulum in the 7 unilateral cases that failed from acetabular roof deficiency we find that the opposite acetabulum was shallow in 3 and undisputedly normal in 4. (These terms are defined in the Wilkinson and Carter paper, 1960.) Shallowness did not persist throughout

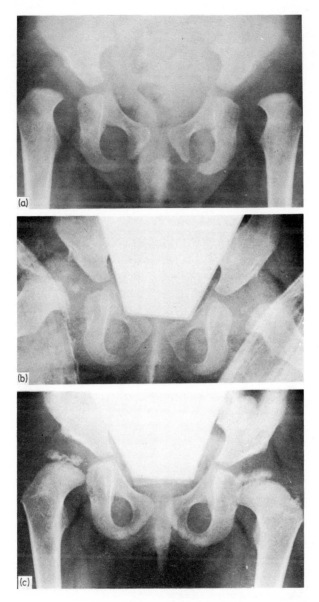

Figure 4.24. Anteroposterior radiographs of bilateral CDH in a girl aged 1 year 5 months (a); The position in Batchelor plaster (b); and the position 2 years later (c). Can a prediction be made of the outcome?

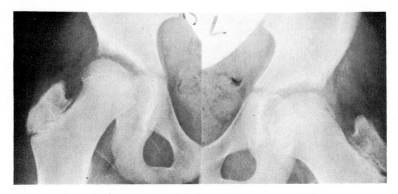

Figure 4.25. Radiograph of the same hips as in Figure 4.24, taken 10 years later. Both function normally but the right hip is graded 'bad' and the left 'good'

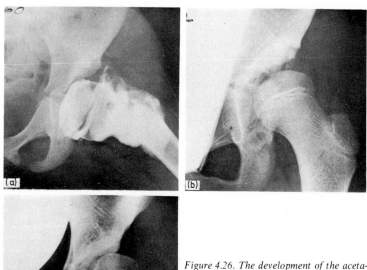

Figure 4.26. The development of the aceta-bulum 5 years (b) and 14 years (c) after an arthrogram (a) gave grounds for believing its ultimate shape would be satisfactory

childhood and in 2 of the 3 so afflicted the opposite side improved as the dislocated side worsened.

Figure 4.24a and *b* show an anteroposterior radiograph of a girl's hips at aged 1 year 5 months, then the position in Batchelor plaster 7 months after convincing manipulative reduction. If an acetabulum will only grow to its genetic potential as Wilkinson and Carter (1960) suggest then we should see here a similar end result on both sides. *Figure 4.24c* shows the hips 2 years later. Ten years after reduction (*Figure 4.25*) there is a normal left hip and a poor right hip. This fact defies explanation. Some who have followed this thesis thus far would say that an arthrogram taken at the time of *Figure 4.24b* would have shown whether the acetabular roof would form or not. But would it?

Figure 4.26a is an anteroposterior arthrogram of a similar hip 7 months after reduction. There is a poor bony acetabular roof but a normal cartilaginous roof is seen. One might expect that ossification would occur in this and give a normal hip 14 years later but this did not happen (*Figure 4.26c*). The girl did not have rotation osteotomy. It is this factor which prevented the acetabular roof from behaving as expected. An arthrogram will show the potential for acetabular roof growth which will only be realized if anteversion is corrected. *Figure 4.27* shows similar arthrographic findings in a girl whose anteversion was corrected by a 90-degree rotation osteotomy. The end result 12 years later shows the expected amount of acetabular development. It is the osteotomy that is important not the arthrogram.

Presence of other abnormalities

Six hips failed in 5 children who had other abnormalities not thought important when hip treatment began. Two had scoliosis associated with poor results in 3 hips. One child had congenital spinal defect and 1 a club foot. The fifth child was mentally retarded.

Thus 6 of the 30 failures did not occur in normal children. Among the 161 good results there was one hip, in a mentally retarded boy. Scoliosis and club-foot were not seen in the good result group but one child with bilateral good results had a cleft palate.

Difficulties in grading

In all papers concerning treatment of CDH the assessment of results is vital. Clearly the nearer this assessment is to skeletal maturity the more accurate. Even at that time, however, great difficulties can arise. The excellent and the poor are usually obvious at this time but the wasteland in between is uncharted. My colleague Mr M. G. H. Smith

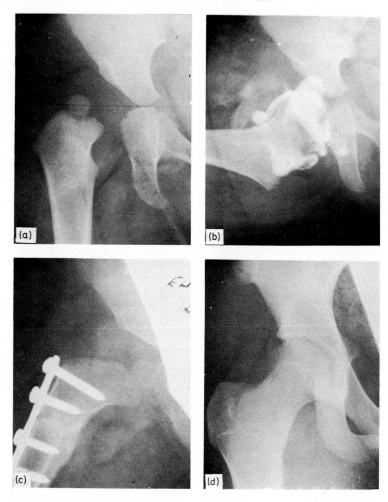

Figure 4.27. Twelve-year result of CDH in a girl aged 15 months. The arthrogram (b) showed acetabular potential which was realized after the rotation osteotomy (c) leading to a normal hip 12 years later (d)

has been an independent assessor of some of the more difficult end-result radiographs in this study. He has used my definitions of good and bad and I extend him my sincere thanks. Validity might be added to this study if I conclude by showing which, in our opinion, are the worst of the good results and the best of the bad.

Figure 4.28 is an anteroposterior radiograph of a girl aged 3 years who presented with limp thought to be due to obesity.

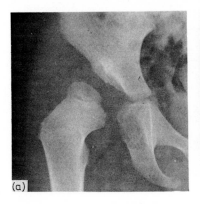
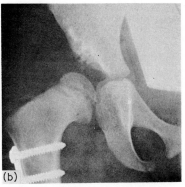

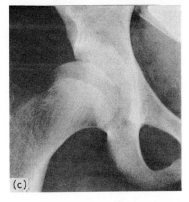

Figure 4.28. The worst of the results graded 'good'. (a) The position on diagnosis; (b) the position 1 year after reduction; and (c) the position 10 years later

Manipulative reduction was followed by the treatment described. The acetabulum was among the worst in the problem hip group. No treatment was given. Ten years after reduction, she was normal. The radiograph placed her in the good group (note the improvement in Shenton's line and see definitions).

Another girl with severe flat feet had her bilateral dislocations reduced at age 2 years. The standard treatment was followed. Five years later, both hips were given a guarded prognosis but 9 years later still, after a full school life, she had joined the Police Cadet Force. She was fully active and pain-free. Radiographs (*Figure 4.29*) showed features that just failed to achieve the good grade.

Conclusions

The rotation osteotomy must be radical. It must produce an appearance of coxa vara where the head is inferior and deep in the acetabulum. This study has not solved the problem of acetabular roof

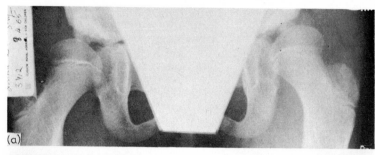

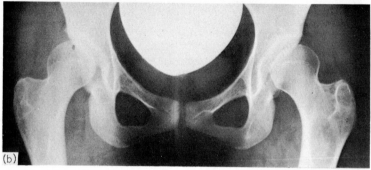

Figure 4.29. The best of the results graded 'bad'. (a) shows the appearances 5 years after reduction of bilateral CDH. (b) shows the hips 14 years after reduction

growth. *Figure 4.15* shows a hip that did badly and yet its appearance is preferable to those shown on *Figure 4.17* and *4.18* which did well.

The good and the bad in the group of 49 problem hips posed similar mechanical problems. The degree of derotation, the fixation of the osteotomy, its after-treatment and follow-up were the same.

And yet 36 of the 49 hips showing features on the PT radiograph suggesting a bad prognosis did well with rotation osteotomy alone. They would perhaps have done equally well in other clinics with acetabuloplasty or innominate osteotomy without rotation osteotomy. Both these latter operations are major undertakings with known and serious complications. They should not be used for all problem hips when the simpler and safer procedure of rotation osteotomy will convert 70 per cent to good results. Their logical place is in the management of the 13 out of 49 (25 per cent), whose acetabular roof shows no response in the year after the end of treatment. If used at this time none will be unnecessary. This thesis is helped by the statement of Mackenzie, Seddon and Trevor (1960) that there was no urgency in performing acetabular surgery, corrective acetabuloplasty being as good as preventive acetabuloplasty. Whether one can afford to wait until actual subluxation occurs or whether one should pre-empt this event is unknown. The evidence suggests that if there is still no osseous support after 1 year of walking, i.e. 1 year and 10 months after reduction there is almost always beginning superior subluxation and a 'bulging' head.

Summary

A programme of treatment that can be expected to give 90 per cent good results in typical congenital dislocation of the hip at between 1 and 4 years of age is described. This includes:

Gentle manipulative reduction and immobilization in a frog plaster just short of full abduction for 3 months or open reduction if indicated by the sensation of manipulation and the radiograph.

One month in an abduction plaster in neutral rotation.

Three months in Batchelor plaster in abduction and full internal rotation if indicated by radiographs.

Rotation osteotomy 7 months after closed reduction or 3 months after open reduction.

Abduction plaster after osteotomy until 10 months post-reduction.

The bad results are more likely to occur in children with other abnormalities and boys will do slightly worse than girls.

The largest single cause of the bad result is failure of the acetabulum to develop. Prognostic difficulty will be found in about 25 per cent of hips when judged at the completion of treatment. If nothing is done to these about 70 per cent will improve spontaneously (provided effective rotation osteotomy has been a part of this treatment).

No single factor explains why some hips fail whereas others appearing similar at the end of treatment succeed.

Acetabular roof development is genetically determined and obeys no rules.

The clinician must decide whether he will master the techniques of this treatment programme, whether he will treat CDH in this age group by open reduction and innominate osteotomy, whether he will perform pelvic surgery on all the problem hips (49 out of 191 or about 25 per cent) or whether he will reserve such surgery for the 25 per cent of the problem hips which in spite of rotation osteotomy fail to show adequate acetabular roof growth. Before embarking on wide use of one or other of the pelvic osteotomies now popular for hips thought likely to subluxate in late childhood we must be able to predict with accuracy which hips will subluxate. This I cannot do.

REFERENCES

Barlow, T. G. (1962). *J. Bone Jt Surg.* **44B**, 292
Campbell, W. C. (1971). *Operative Orthopaedics* (5th edn). Edited by A. H. Crenshaw. 2 vols. St. Louis; C. V. Mosby
Chiari, K. (1955). *Z. Orthop.* **87**, 14
Finlay, H. V. L., Maudesley, R. H. and Busfield, P. I. (1967). *Br. med. J.* **4**, 377
Howarth, M. B. (1935). *J. Bone Jt Surg.* **17**, 945
MacKenzie, I. G. (1972). *J. Bone Jt Surg.* **54B**, 18
— Seddon, H. J. and Trevor, D. (1960). *J. Bone Jt Surg.* **42B**, 689
Mitchell, G. P. (1972). *J. Bone Jt Surg.* **54B**, 4
Müller, G. M. and Seddon, H. J. (1953). *J. Bone Jt Surg.* **35B**, 342
Ortolani, M. (1937). *Paed. Napoli* **45**, 129
Pemberton, P. A. (1961). *J. Bone Jt Surg.* **40A**, 724
Record, R. G. and Edwards, J. H. (1958). *Br. J. prev. soc. Med.* **12**, 8
Salter, R. B. (1961). *J. Bone Jt Surg.* **43B**, 518
— and Dubos, J. P. (1974). *Clin. Orthop.* **98**, 72
— and Kostuik, J. (1969). *Can. J. Surg.* **12**, 44
Severin, E. (1941). *Acta chir. scand.* **84**, (Suppl. 63)
Sharrard, W. J. W. (1972). *Paediatric Orthopaedics and Fractures.* London; Backwell
Smith, W. S., Badgley, C. E., Orwig, J. B. and Harper, J. M. (1968). *J. Bone Jt Surg.* **50A**, 1081
Solomon, L. (1973). *J. Bone Jt Surg.* **55B**, 438
Somerville, E. W. (1953). *J. Bone Jt Surg.* **35B**, 363
— (1974). Personal communication
— and Scott, J. C. (1957). *J. Bone Jt Surg.* **39B**, 623
Stanisavljevic, S. (1964). *Congenital Hip Pathology in Newborn.* Baltimore; Waverly
Van Rosen, S. (1962). *J. Bone Jt Surg.* **44B**, 284
Wiberg, G. (1939). *Acta chir. scand.* **83**, (Suppl. 58)
Wilkinson, J. A. and Carter, C. (1960). *J. Bone Jt Surg.* **42B**, 669

5 Observations on Infantile Idiopathic Scoliosis

The Milwaukee brace has an unassailable position in the management of progressive infantile idiopathic scoliosis. James (1967) described improvement of more than 5 degrees in 21 out of 25 children whose scoliosis began before age 10 years and who were known to be worsening before the brace was applied. More recently James (1974) spoke of his experience of 120 children with infantile idiopathic scoliosis. Ninety had undergone spontaneous resolution by their sixth year. Of the other 30, all destined for serious deformity, 14 were following the programme of plaster correction, followed by Milwaukee bracing, when applicable, ending with spinal fusion, 6 had completed the treatment and 8 more were awaiting fusion. In the 6 children whose treatment was complete the final radiograph in 5 showed a smaller angle of scoliosis than on their original radiograph. Another group of 10 scoliotic curves behaved differently in that with plaster correction and bracing alone they disappeared. Study of the original radiographs of these children by Mehta's method (1972) suggested that they might have been in the group of resolving curves.

In spite of flirtations with convex side rib fusions, vertebral body stapling, epiphysiodesis and various internal metallic distraction devices, the Milwaukee brace remains the most reliable and effective treatment for curves known to have a bad prognosis. Its success depends on acceptability and accurate construction. The moulded leather pelvic girdle has to exaggerate the child's waist and cannot be constructed without an original negative plaster cast. It is thus essential to have a patient with a waist and one who will co-operate with the making of this cast. I find these qualities rare under the age of 5 years. What, then, can be done for a child with a worsening infantile idiopathic curve at age 2 years? James treats such a child with a hinging Risser jacket to correct the curve followed by the repeated application of plaster jackets renewed as the child grows, until a brace can be made. As this period can be as long as 3 years, it seemed wise to try a different kind of plaster jacket used for 3 months in every 12 to hold the curve until the child was old enough for a Milwaukee brace.

Clearly the first problem is the distinction between resolving and progressive curves, which appear identical at the time of diagnosis. It has been shown that 90 per cent of infantile idiopathic thoracic curves are resolving (Lloyd-Roberts and Pilcher, 1965). They are usually less than 20 degrees when first seen and disappear slowly by age 5 years. The 10 per cent which are progressive tend to be more than 20 degrees on diagnosis and tend to have a greater incidence of associated developmental anomaly (Conner, 1969). Other radiological characteristics have been discovered by Mehta (1972). She studied 138 case records from a group of 361 children who attended the Royal National Orthopaedic Hospital, London. From this group she selected retrospectively 46 infantile idiopathic curves which resolved and 40 which progressed. Studying the original anteroposterior radiographs of these children she found that if the head of the rib on the convex side overlapped the superolateral corner of the apical vertebra the curve was likely to be progressive. She also drew in the rib vertebra angle on both sides of the curve and found that the difference between the concave side and the convex side measured the droop of the convex side ribs. This RVAD (rib vertebra angle difference) was 20 degrees or more in curves destined to progress and was found to increase with time. These conclusions of Mehta's are based upon drawing lines on radiographic shadows of ribs and vertebrae of small infants (only 2 of the 46 resolving cases were over 16 months of age). These lines must surely be influenced by positioning and respiration (see Catterall, 1970, 'Ex umbris eruditio').

In Glasgow our predictions from original radiographs of infantile scoliosis have been less accurate. In 44 children the RVAD has been measured by a consultant radiologist ignorant of the outcome and using Mehta's criteria the correlation was 60 per cent (Conner and Sweet, 1974). We see no urgent need to distinguish the two groups in the first year of life. One can afford to wait because treatment is seldom offered until age 2 years. Then the presence of fixed rotation with a pronounced rib hump and of compensatory curves above and below a primary thoracic curve seen to worsen to 35 degrees or more indicate a bad prognosis and demand treatment.

THE LATERAL SUSPENSION JACKET

Whatever the underlying cause of scoliosis, a prominent element is soft-tissue contracture on the concave side. If this were not present it would easily be possible to straighten the spine. This contracture may lie at the sides of the rotated bodies or at any point lateral to this. The progression of the curve if left untreated suggests that this tissue is relatively inextensible and does not grow as does normal tissue. The aims of the Risser techniques and the Milwaukee brace are to stretch this tissue and thus abolish as far as is possible its tethering effects. It follows, therefore, that the most effective plaster jacket will be one which stretches the tissues in the concavity as much as possible. Local pressure on the convexity is not as good as direct stretch on the concavity. The force to apply is that of gravity and to be maximally effective it must operate without muscle tone

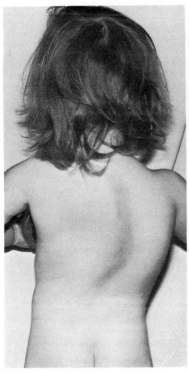

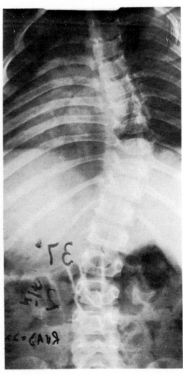

Figure 5.1. Infantile idiopathic scoliosis of progressive type in a girl aged 2 years 4 months

Figure 5.2 Anteroposterior radiograph

opposing it. With these principles in mind a technique was evolved in 1969 whose early results can now be reported.

Figures 5.1 and *5.2* show the clinical and radiological features of a girl aged 2 years 4 months. An earlier x-ray taken at age 2 years had shown an idiopathic thoracic scoliosis of 30 degrees. We had seen the curve worsen and the child develop pronounced rotation in the 4-month period of observation. The RVAD was 22 degrees on the film shown and 18 degrees on

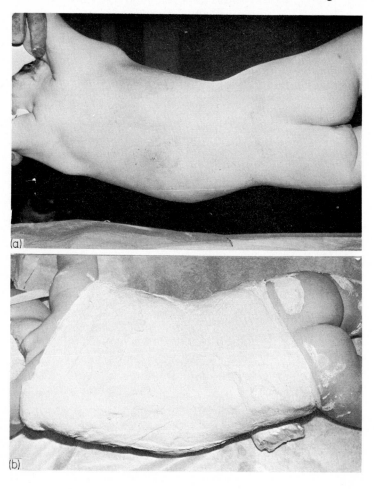

Figure 5.3. (a) The child is suspended left side down thus allowing gravity to open the concavity. (b) The plaster jacket is completed. Note felt pads in the left axilla and groin

film taken 4 months previously. These were accepted as criteria suggesting a progressive deformity. The curve was convex to the right of 37 degrees with the apex at T9.

Under general anaesthesia (Ketalar is ideal for this) she was

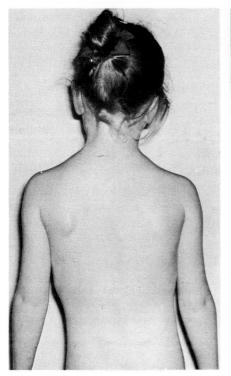

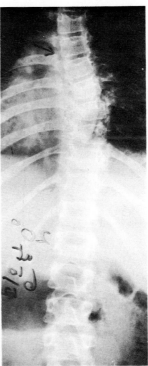

Figure 5.4. The same girl as in Figure 5.1 at age 6 years 10 months

Figure 5.5. Anteroposterior radiograph at age 6 years 10 months

turned left side down and suspended by supports under the left thigh and the left arm. The whole trunk was allowed to sag to the position shown (*Figure 5.3a*), thus opening up the concavity of the curve.

With felt padding in the axillae and over the iliac crests the plaster jacket was applied (*Figure 5.3b*), fitting closely into the left axilla.

Her efforts to bring the left arm to her side caused leverage over the smooth felt pad upon the structures in the concavity of her curve. The procedure was repeated 1 month and 2 months later. After 3 months all plaster was abandoned. A further three jackets were applied in her third year and again in her fourth year. In each case she had the 3 winter months in plaster, and the other 9 free. After the third set of jackets, i.e. at age $4\frac{1}{2}$ years, radiographs showed a curve of 21 degrees, the rib hump had improved and it was decided to withhold the Milwaukee brace until there was evidence of deterioration again. This did not occur, and at age 6 years and 10 months she had maintained the correction achieved. The clinical and radiological appearances at that time are as shown in *Figure 5.4* and *Figure 5.5*.

The second girl in whom this technique was used had an infantile idiopathic curve of 56 degrees convex to the right apex T11 at age 4 years (*Figure 5.6a*). Her older sister also had idiopathic thoracic scoliosis. She was treated in two series of tilt jackets, each lasting 3 months. *Figure 5.6b* shows the correction achieved during the first series of jackets. At age 6 years she was left free. The spine was straighter, this position was maintained and now at age 11 years (*Figure 5.7*) she is normal.

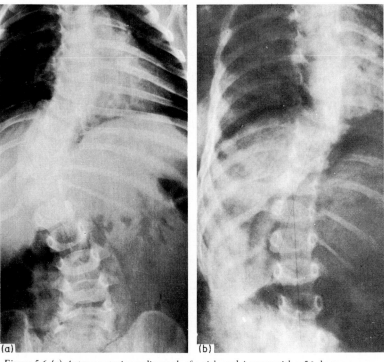

(a)   (b)

Figure 5.6. (a) Anteroposterior radiograph of a girl aged 4 years with a 56-degree curve.
(b) Radiograph of the same spine after application of the tilt jacket

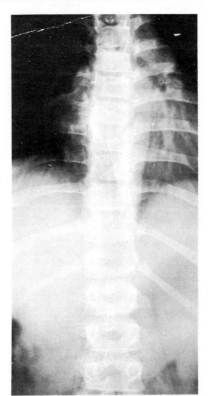

Figure 5.7. Anteroposterior radiograph at age 9 years of the same girl as in Figure 5.6

Whilst this technique was intended as a prelude to Milwaukee-brace treatment, in neither of these first two cases was this necessary. Thus either two idiopathic curves were misdiagnosed as progressive and unnecessarily treated or the lateral suspension jacket described has, by stretching the tissues in the concavity, created conditions leading to resolution of the curve.

The next figures show the amount of correction that is possible in severe curves in the very young. *Figure 5.8a* shows an idiopathic curve of 44 degrees at 11 months of age. She was treated by three series of jackets for the 3 winter months. *Figure 5.8b* shows the spine at age 4 years in the last jacket. Although relapse occurs in the annual 9 months of freedom, it is possible on each occasion to get back to an acceptable position. She is now awaiting development of the physical contours that make a Milwaukee brace effective.

There have been no complications in any patient so treated. The technique is recommended to all those who like me look upon the

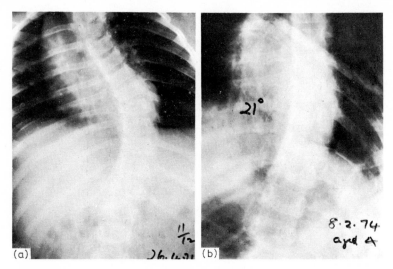

Figure 5.8. (a) Anteroposterior radiograph of the spine of a girl aged 11 months with a 44-degree curve. (b) The same spine at age 4 years. The curve has been held

severe progressive idiopathic curve in the young infant as one of the most difficult problems in orthopaedics.

REFERENCES

Catterall, R. C. F. (1970). *J. Bone Jt Surg.* **50B,** 455
Conner, A. N. (1969). *J. Bone Jt Surg.* **51B,** 711
— and Sweet, E. (1974). Personal communication
James, J. I. P. (1951). *J. Bone Jt Surg.* **33B,** 399
— (1967). *Scoliosis.* Edinburgh; Livingstone
— (1974). *J. Bone Jt Surg.* **56B,** 566
Lloyd-Roberts, G. C. and Pilcher, M. F. (1965). *J. Bone Jt Surg.* **47B,** 520
Mehta, M. H. (1972). *J. Bone Jt Surg.* **54B,** 230

6 On the Question of Whether to Treat, and if so, When

Whilst attempting to treat apparently amenable deformities over the years I have been struck by the reasonableness of the result when my efforts either totally failed or were declined. Maturity makes failure less easy to bear and danger less acceptable. This chapter looks at a variety of children's orthopaedic lesions where these lessons have been learned. There are some which I now do not treat at all and others where the right timing of treatment increases the chance of success and lessens danger. As elsewhere in paediatrics we must know what the condition would be like if the child's mother had consulted us 10 or 15 years hence. In conditions where we have this knowledge we can look more critically at some of the ingenious operations designed to correct these conditions, particularly those whose published follow-up is short. The importance of knowledge of natural history is exemplified by considering congenital short-leg.

Congenital absence of the fibula and fifth ray of the foot is often seen with anterior tibial bowing and a characteristic skin blemish over the tibia. This compound deformity will lead to a shortening of 4 inches (10 cm) or more by skeletal maturity. Ingenious and radical operations designed for its correction can only be judged if there is a long-term follow-up. Serafin (1967) reports results on 3 children with a follow-up of 17 to 27 months. The wisest treatment is a Syme-type amputation performed at age 2 years. In one patient, however, this advice was declined and it was therefore possible to follow the natural history from infancy to maturity without treatment. *Figure 6.1a* shows the lower legs of a boy aged 13 days. The only treatment

given was to the left talipes equinovarus. The legs at age 16 years
are shown in *Figure 6.1b*. Although equinovalgus had developed in
the right leg and also hallux valgus the function was good. In another
boy with congenital absence of the fibula and fifth ray of the foot
(*Figure 6.2a*) the valgus was corrected by open radical excision of
the fascial remnant of the fibula, making possible the placing of the
foot under the tibia. This position was held for 2 years in plaster
and no further treatment given. At age 17 years the leg was 4 inches

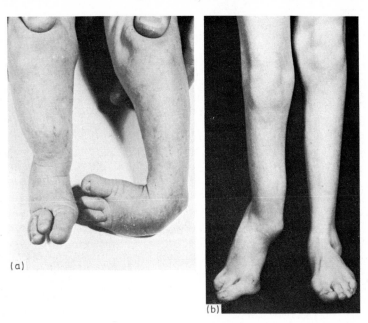

(a)

(b)

*Figure 6.1. (a) The lower legs of a boy aged 13 days. (b) The same legs at age 16 years.
Only the left foot was treated.*

(10 cm) short but the function was good (*Figure 6.2b*). I have not
had sufficient success with leg lengthening operations in congenitally
short tibiae to recommend this operation. Step osteotomy of the tibia
and gradual elongation by skeletal traction can be relied upon to
give 2-inch (5-cm) lengthening without complications in post-para-
lytic shortening but not, in my hands, in congenital shortening. In
girls the amputation advised is the transtarsal operation of Boyd (with
a long plantar flap) (*Figure 6.3*). This is preferred to the Syme or
below-knee operation because of the length saved. Equinus of the
stump will occur but is not troublesome. A prosthesis with no above-
knee attachment can be fitted and will resemble a fashion boot.

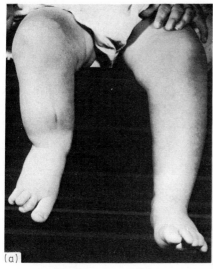

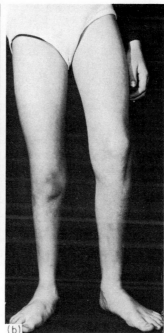

Figure 6.2. Seventeen-year result of treating congenital absence of the fibula by soft-tissue surgery

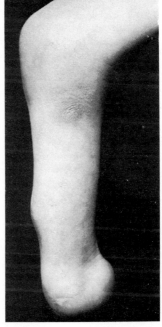

Figure 6.3. The stump 6 years after transtarsal amputation

LESIONS TO BE LEFT ALONE

Some familiarity with long-term follow-up has led me to avoid and dissuade others from operations designed to treat most children afflicted with the following conditions.

Congenital contracture of fingers

Campylodactyly or congenital contracture of the fifth finger affects girls and like curling toe shows a disparity between the length of the bones and of the soft tissues, the latter being too short to allow the joints to be fully extended. All tissues on the flexor aspect of the digit are tight. Z-plasty of the flexor skin attacks but one element of a complex deformity. I have looked at the more ambitious operations described by other writers including flexor tendon transplant to the extensor surface (Sharrard, 1971) and shortening of the proximal phalanx (Oldfield, 1955) but have realized that the untreated deformity does not get worse. Totally untreated, the hand is capable of any activity, including piano playing. The ultimate deformity is only noticed on rare occasions when an attempt is made fully to extend the fingers. The present 'leave alone' attitude results from disappointment with radical surgery. Open anterior division of tight tissues fixing the interphalangeal (IP) joint in extension with a wire has failed and on one occasion the 'open palm' technique giving such good results in adult Dupuytren's contracture has been used. Through a transverse incision all tight tissues were divided including the whole of the flexor tendon sheath. The only anterior structures left intact were the flexor tendons and the neurovascular bundles. The finger was straightened, leaving a half-inch gap in the anterior skin. Although splinted straight the wound healed in 4 weeks but thereafter the finger gradually flexed again to its pre-operative state. *Figure 6.4* shows this recurrence 6 months after the radical operation. Congenital contractures, unlike scar contractures, do not seem amenable to the 'open palm' technique.

Curled fingers

It is normal for infants to hold their fingers clenched for the first 2 months of life. Thereafter the clenched fist posture usually relaxes requiring less pressure as months advance. If there are deep flexor creases on the flexor aspect recovery, even with apparent persistent flexion at 6 months of age, will occur. If there are no skin creases each finger will behave as described in the previous paragraph. They will extend a little more as years pass—passive stretching may be useful—and at age 12 years there will be good function and a passable appearance.

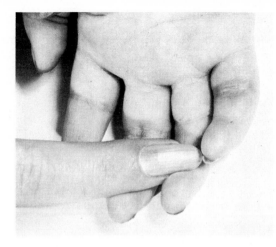

Figure 6.4. Recurrence of contracture after open-palm technique

Sprengel's shoulder

This deformity gives the impression that open division of the tight structures tethering the scapula to the spinous processes will allow descent and consequent improved function and appearance. The technique of Green (1957) has been used twice and augmented by fixing the lowered scapula to a short plaster hip spica with a subcutaneous wire. In both cases the success achieved has been lost within a year with reversion to the same position as in the pre-operative state. Complex congenital deformities like this cannot be cured by surgical attention to only one element of the deformity. I have not known function or appearance to worsen in untreated cases.

Pigeon chest

Pectus excavatus shows in my experience a tendency to spontaneous improvement. Whilst not rare in young boys conspicuous deformity was not seen in 2 years of examining teenage Royal Air Force recruits. *Figure 6.5a* shows a depression of the left anterior ribs of a boy aged 3 years whose appearance caused concern. *Figure 6.5b* shows the same boy 15 years later. No treatment except deep breathing exercises had been given. The radical operations described for this condition do not seem justified.

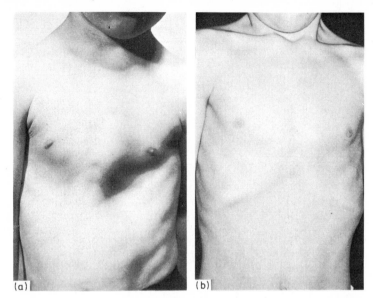

Figure 6.5. (a) Pectus excavatus in a boy aged 3 years. (b) The same boy at age 18 years

Congenital synostosis of the forearm

Here the forearm is locked in the position of slight pronation. Because of this fortunate circumstance disability is trivial. Surgery designed to create a radio-ulna pseudarthrosis with or without fascial interposition and with or without repeated manipulation has always failed in my hands.

Congenital instability of the knee

This congenital deformity is seen following breech delivery with extended legs. There is commonly an additional hip or foot deformity. In the neonatal period the knee dislocation can be successfully reduced and splinted in flexion. If this chance is missed the decision whether to embark upon a radical extensor muscle lengthening and open reduction of the knee has to be made. This procedure (Curtis and Fisher, 1969) has been disappointing in my hands. In 2 such children fibrous ankylosis of the knee has developed which required arthrodesis in later childhood. The disability of untreated anterior displacement of the tibia is not severe. The quadriceps lengthen a little with time. Pain and lateral instability do not develop. *Figure 6.6* shows the condition of the left knee of a girl at 2 months old and at 14 years old. In spite of recurrent subluxation occurring at every step her knee is painless and fully mobile.

No permanent success has resulted from surgical management of recurrent lateral dislocation of the patella where there is no knock-knee deformity. In this condition the patellae are high, small and globular. On each knee flexion they slip over the lateral edge of the lower femur as if pulled by tight bands in the fascia lata. If there is significant knock-knee the Hauser operation (1938) is successful

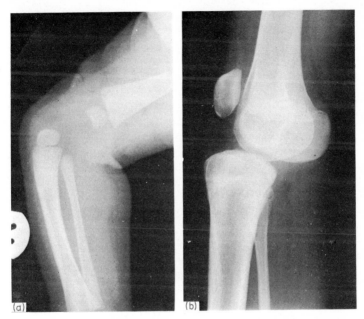

Figure 6.6. Lateral radiographs of the knee of a girl aged 2 months (a) and 14 years (b) with untreated instability of the knee joint

but the disability from lateral dislocation of the patella in a straight leg is trivial and its correction does not justify the serious complications that can result from interference of upper tibial growth.

Post-infective dislocation of the hip

Others have reported success following open reduction after dislocation of the hip from pyogenic arthritis of infancy. In spite of many attempts I have been pleased with none. The nearest to success was a girl aged 2 years whose neck of femur was not totally destroyed by the pyogenic arthritis in the neonatal period. An open reduction

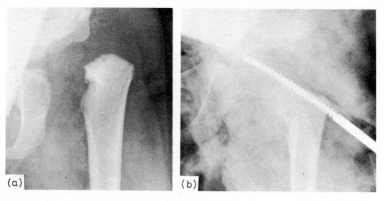

Figure 6.7. Dislocation of the hip secondary to suppurative arthritis of infancy (a). Open reduction with fixation of the hip in a reduced position (b). The operation failed

was performed and the stump of the neck held into the deepened acetabulum after extensive excision of scar tissue by inserting a malleable screw up the neck into the acetabular floor—this step was necessary to hold reduction. The screw was removed at 3 months when rotation osteotomy was performed (*Figure 6.7*). One year later the femoral neck stump moved laterally and proximally giving a result no better than those offered by no treatment.

Other hip lesions

This compilation of lesions where energetic treatment has proved disappointing must include meningomyelocele where the paralysis includes the first lumbar segment. Infants so afflicted often have severe spinal deformity which renders splintage for their totally paralysed legs so inhibiting that wheelchair life is preferable, and thus surgically corrected feet and knees are of no importance.

'Pre-natal' bilateral congenital dislocation of hips in boys has been badly managed on many occasions. The baby has radiological evidence of false acetabuli soon after birth and clinical examination gives negative Ortolani signs because of the irreducibility of the hips. In some there is limitation of abduction of the hips due to tight perineal skin. This feature is an absolute contra-indication to treatment. In its presence the type of reduction required is a very extensive open reduction of each hip followed by rotation osteotomy if both open reductions achieve success. Thus embarking on treatment necessitates four operations, all of which have to be successful if the ultimate result is to be preferable to the untreated state. Success on one side and failure on the other produces a limb length

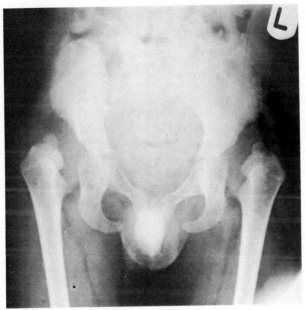

Figure 6.8. Radiograph of a boy aged 5 years with 'pre-natal' congenital dislocation of the hips, wisely left untreated

difference which was not present before. The end result of withholding treatment is a rolling gait but excellent function.

Figure 6.8 is a radiograph of a boy aged 5 years with bilateral 'pre-natal' dislocation of the hips. He was thin, firm and wiry, as is typical of teratological dislocation, with limited abduction and rotation. No treatment was given.

'Osteochondritis'

Minor irregularities of ossification of the femoral head with or without symptoms and signs have been shown to clear just as quickly and completely in children under age 4 years without treatment as with treatment. These irregularities are often labelled 'Perthes' disease' and treated accordingly. It is possible to distinguish the irregularity (*Figure 6.9a*) from the genuine avascular, squashed, dense epiphysis associated with thigh-wasting and loss of abduction essential for the diagnosis of Perthes' disease. *Figure 6.9b* shows the same hip 7 years later following no treatment.

Similar ossific irregularities appear in the heel (Sever's disease) and in the tarsal navicular (Kohler's disease). These conditions

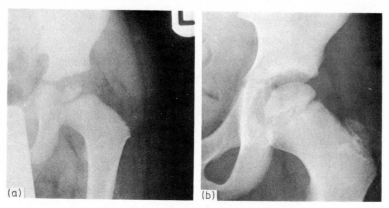

Figure 6.9. Irregular mineralization—not Perthes' disease. (a) The hip at age 3 years. (b) The same hip at age 10 years without treatment

appear to resolve completely within 6 months and need not be treated.

LESIONS WHERE TIMING OF TREATMENT IS IMPORTANT

Orthopaedic lesions to be treated at birth

Congenital dislocation of the hip giving a positive 'clunk' test on day 1 and again on day 7 in execution of which the fatty tissue shakes should be splinted for 3 months in abduction on a divaricator splint. Other physical signs in the hip of the newborn, including evidence of irreducible dislocation, should not be treated at this stage.

Congenital talipes equinovarus and congenital metatarsus varus in which the metatarsal bases are laterally displaced should have repeated, strong manipulations and splintage. The soft-tissue contracture producing these deformities must be overcome before there is significant change in the shape of the tarsal bones. If attention is paid to the direction of the forces applied to the deformed child's foot spurious corrections will not be so frequent (*Figure 6.10*).

Excision and repair of lumbar meningomyelocele where there is evidence of motor innervation of at least the first lumbar spinal segment, i.e. flexed hips indicating psoas function, are easier when performed in the first 24 hours of life. The peripheral deformities of lumbar meningocele should be treated by passive exercises and not splintage. All other lower motor neurone lesions present at birth should be treated.

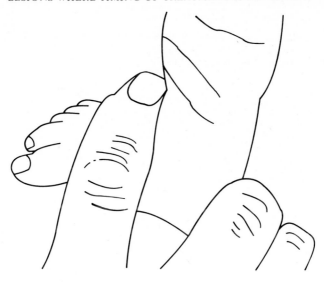

Figure 6.10. Manipulation of congenital club-foot. The grip used to avoid spurious correction. The thumb pushes the anterior tarsus upwards as the middle finger pulls the posterior tarsus downwards

Congenital flat foot—vertical talus

The term 'congenital flat foot' should be reserved for the deformity present at birth (*Figure 6.11*), where the calcaneus is in equinus, the medial border and medial longitudinal arch are convex and where the first metatarsal is extended on the tarsus. Sometimes in addition there is distension of the medial skin by the vertical disposition of the talus. The foot looks nothing like a normal foot and its complex deformity will persist if not treated, leading to a valgus foot with a callosity over the talar head. No lesser degree of deformity should be included in this 'vertical talus syndrome'.

Correction must be achieved in the first 6 months of life. The foot is plantar-flexed forcibly and encased in plaster. This is repeated with suitable wedging until the correct anatomical relationships have been restored. The long axis of the talus must be in line with the long axis of the first metatarsal (*Figure 6.12a*). The foot is then held in this position for 6 months. The plaster is removed and walking encouraged. If the foot remains in tight equinus the tendo Achilles has to be lengthened and if necessary a posterior capsulotomy of the ankle performed to allow the foot to become plantigrade without the calcaneus reverting to its equinus position. Two out of 3 will correct spontaneously without any posterior foot operation. *Figure 6.12b* is a radiograph of the same foot 5 years after correction.

Corrections beginning after weight-bearing has started are

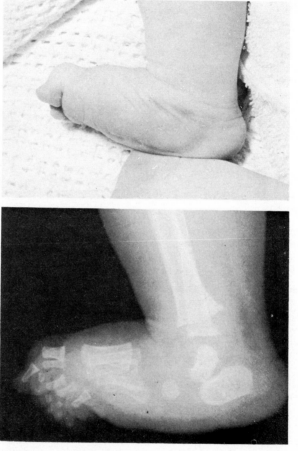

Figure 6.11. The classic clinical and radiological features of congenital flat foot (vertical talus)

doomed to failure. Tendon transplants to the neck of the talus, reefing the medial capsule, shortening of the plantar fascia and excision of the navicular have been tried separately and in combination without success. Such feet remain flat and valgus and are best encased in shoes with a sponge-rubber Whitman brace, an outside iron and

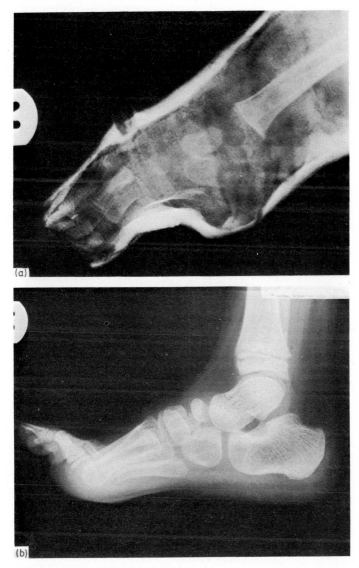

Figure 6.12. (a) *The same foot as in Figure 6.11, after serial plasters with wedging.* (b) *The same foot at age 5 years*

short, inside T-strap. I can recall no case in children's orthopaedics where operative shortening of a ligament has achieved its purpose.

Orthopaedic lesions to be treated after 1 year of age

Under this heading are lesions which can be treated as soon as diagnosed but where my results have been better when this treatment has been delayed.

Irreducible 'pre-natal' dislocation of the hips, if unilateral in boys or bilateral in girls, gives better ultimate results if, when neonatal reduction fails, the parents exercise the affected hip and definitive reduction by open operation is carried out in the second year of life.

The management of neonatal foot deformities due to congenital lumbar spine lesions by splintage or plaster can be disastrous. The pressure required to hold equinovarus feet in the corrected position cannot be tolerated by anaesthetic skin, plasters change position and pressure sores are common. Better long-term results are achieved by encouraging passive movements of all joints of the lower limbs after surgical excision of the meningocele. These movements may prevent contractures and dislocation of the hip. They will not correct deformed feet. This correction can be better achieved in the second year of life at the time when lower limb bracing to facilitate standing is best carried out. I have not known calipers with pelvic band or jacket to be of any real use to any child under age 2 years.

Amputations of accessory fingers and toes and amputations of grossly deformed feet associated with congenital absence of the tibia should be carried out in the second year of life. Such seemingly mutilating operations require for their success parents who have become convinced of their necessity. In children's orthopaedics there are parents as well as patients to consider. On the other hand, waiting too long before the definitive step can limit the child's activities, attract ridicule or foster embarrassment. Radical ablative procedures are therefore performed at around the first birthday leaving the older child with no memory of the original deformity or of the stay in hospital.

Leaving lesions treatable when diagnosed until after the first birthday has the advantage of making the operation and its subsequent splintage easier because the parts are bigger. Thus operations for trigger thumb can produce 100 per cent successful results when performed in the second year. Open operation for CDH should not be performed earlier than this. Accurate identification of tissues is easier when their shape, size and texture approaches that with which the surgeon is familiar. This argument applies with force to relapsed club-foot. Early forceful and repeated manipulations in the first months of life will correct and render flat almost any twisted foot. Those where no progress is being made should have open elongation of the tendo calcaneus which lowers the heel and enables manipulations to continue effectively. More extensive surgery should be delayed. The relapse rate in club-foot is 50 per cent occurring in the second year of life. Radical medial release operations should be delayed for these relapsed feet until the second year or later. Borderline cases can be managed by repeated manipulations and plaster

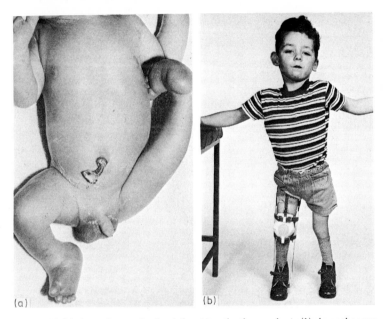

Figure 6.13. (a) shows the complex leg deformities of arthrogryphosis. (b) shows the same boy at age 4 years. Corrections were performed at age 3 years

fixation until the tissues are big enough to make the operation an exact and complete excision of tight pathological tissue and a careful lengthening of tendons. If performed late in the second year of life there will be fewer undercorrections through inability to excise totally what has to be removed and fewer overcorrections by avoidance of operative mistakes. In complex lower limb deformities associated with meningomyelocele or arthrogryphosis it is common to find the well-intentioned, early, limb operations have to be repeated in later childhood. It is impossible to apply an effective padded plaster to a tapering limb unless the foot deformity can be completely corrected to a right-angled position—the plaster will slip off. There will be relapse of the foot deformity unless weight-bearing and boot and caliper splintage can hold the correction the operation has achieved. For these reasons surgical corrections are better delayed until age 2 years or more. The baby shown in *Figure 6.13a* received open correction of the right knee and extensive medial release operations of the feet in the first 6 months of life. He did not stand until age 3 years by which time all three operations had to be repeated because of relapse. At age 3 years we had the benefit of his co-operation as well as the advantage of bigger limbs (*Figure 6.13b*).

Operations to be performed between age 3 and 5 years

Where the patient's co-operation is necessary for a good result operation should be delayed, if possible, until this age period. Open correction of muscular torticollis, z-plasty of skin contractures and elongation of the tendo achilles for spastic equinus fall into this group.

Congenital adduction of the fifth toe and syndactyly of fingers will give better results if operative correction can be delayed until age 4–5 years.

REFERENCES

Curtis, B. H. and Fisher, R. L. (1969). *J. Bone Jt Surg.* **51A**, 255
Green, W. T. (1957). *J. Bone Jt Surg.* **39A**, 1439
Hauser, E. D. W. (1938). *Surgery Gynec. Obstet.* **66**, 199
Oldfield, M. C. (1955). *Br. J. plast. Surg.* **8**, 312
Serafin, J. (1967). *J. Bone Jt Surg.* **49B**, 59
Sharrard, W. J. W. (1971). *Paediatric Orthopaedics and Fractures.* Oxford; Blackwell

Index